PON

More praise for *The Breast Cancer Book*,
by Ruth H. Grobstein, M.D., Ph.D.

"This is an easy-to-read, very comprehensive book that will answer
any question a woman might have about approaching a diagnosis
of breast cancer."—Vincent T. Devita, M.D., coeditor of *Cancer:
Principles and Practice of Oncology*

"Dr. Ruth Grobstein's book *The Breast Cancer Book* is like having
the most qualified doctor at your bedside answering your questions."
—Hinda Gould Rosenthal, president of the Richard and Hinda
Rosenthal Foundation and trustee of The Yale Cancer Center

"Dr. Grobstein has managed to combine the technical scientific
knowledge with the laypersons' comprehension. The book should be
the readable encyclopedia for all whose life comes in contact with
cancer."—Audrey Geisel, Dr. Seuss Enterprises

"When I was told I had breast cancer I was terrified. If *The Breast
Cancer Book* had been available for me to read prior to my diagnosis
many of my worst fears would have been greatly alleviated. This book
should be required reading for all high school seniors."—Jeanne
Jones, author, consultant, and syndicated columnist

"Dr. Grobstein is a caring, expert oncologist who listens carefully
to her patients. This book is evidence of her understanding what
patients, their friends, and their family want to know."—Dr. Samuel
Hellman, coeditor of *Cancer: Principles and Practice of Oncology*

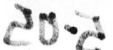

"A diagnosis of breast cancer is one of the most feared messages that a woman can receive. Knowledge is power, and the sage advice provided by the author, Dr. Ruth Grobstein, in this insightful book will be invaluable to all those women who are faced with making difficult decisions about their treatment options and also to individuals who seek expert information for their loved ones about this complex subject."—Margaret Foti, Ph.D., M.D. (hc), CEO, American Association for Cancer Research

"If you or a loved one have been threatened with breast cancer, I urge you to run to the nearest bookstore and buy this book—it might well prove to be life saving. I have sent dozens of my friends to Dr. Ruth Grobstein, and without exception, they have called or written to thank me for sending them to Ruth, for her advice made all the difference as they regained confidence and faith in the future."
—Deborah Szelsky, Founder, Golden Door and Rancho La Puerta

The Breast Cancer Book

Yale University Press Health & Wellness

A Yale University Press Health & Wellness book is an authoritative, accessible source of information on a health-related topic. It may provide guidance to help you lead a healthy life, examine your treatment options for a specific condition or disease, situate a healthcare issue in the context of your life as a whole, or address questions or concerns that linger after visits to your healthcare provider.

Ruth H. Grobstein, M.D., Ph.D., *The Breast Cancer Book: What You Need to Know to Make Informed Decisions*

James W. Hicks, M.D., *Fifty Signs of Mental Illness: A Guide to Understanding Mental Health*

Mary Jane Minkin, M.D., and Carol V. Wright, Ph.D., *A Woman's Guide to Menopause and Perimenopause*

Mary Jane Minkin, M.D., and Carol V. Wright, Ph.D., *A Woman's Guide to Sexual Health*

Catherine M. Poole, with DuPont Guerry IV, M.D., *Melanoma: Prevention, Detection, and Treatment*, 2nd ed.

The Breast Cancer Book

What You Need to Know to Make Informed Decisions

Ruth H. Grobstein, M.D., Ph.D.

Yale University Press New Haven & London

The information and suggestions in this book are not intended to replace the services of your physician or caregiver. Because each person and each medical situation is unique, you should consult your own physician to get answers to your personal questions, to evaluate any symptoms you may have, or to receive suggestions on appropriate medications.

The author has attempted to make this book as accurate and up to date as possible, but it may nevertheless contain errors, omissions, or material that is out of date at the time you read it. Neither the author nor the publisher has any legal responsibility or liability for errors, omissions, out-of-date material, or the reader's application of the medical information or advice contained in this book.

Designed by Rebecca Gibb. Set in Scala type by BW&A Books, Inc.
Printed in the United States of America.

Library of Congress Cataloging-in-Publication Data
Grobstein, Ruth H.
The breast cancer book : what you need to know to make informed decisions /
Ruth H. Grobstein.
     p. cm.
ISBN 0-300-10413-8 (pbk. : alk. paper)
1. Breast—Cancer—Popular works. I. Title.
RC280.B8G737 2005
616.99'449—dc22   2004059861

A catalogue record for this book is available from the British Library. The paper in this book meets the guidelines for permanence and durability of the Committee on Production Guidelines for Book Longevity of the Council on Library Resources.

10 9 8 7 6 5 4 3 2 1

For all my patients, who taught me the importance of listening

Contents

List of Resources 159

Tear-out decision trees appear at the end of the book.

Foreword

Breast cancer—few words carry as much fear. In the United States alone, one out of every seven women will be diagnosed with breast cancer if all live their full life span. This sobering statistic, however, is only part of the story.

Today, more women than ever before are surviving their initial diagnosis—with the help of early screening and detection. And research is offering new hope for effective treatments that attack the tumor without destroying surrounding tissue. In fact, the scientific community believes that we are at a crossroads for conquering this disease.

In addition to scientific and medical advances, another factor will play a major role in this battle—the informed patient. As the saying goes, knowledge is power. When it comes to an illness such as breast cancer, this is more than just a saying. Knowledge may well be the difference between life and death. It is not only power, but it can also help overcome fear—the natural fear that every cancer patient has and the associated fear felt by family members and close friends.

The Breast Cancer Book: What You Need to Know to Make Informed Decisions, written by Ruth H. Grobstein, M.D., Ph.D., represents an important new source of fundamental information that anyone facing breast cancer—whether woman or man—should read. Also, anyone who is worried about breast cancer, or simply wants more information about the subject, will gain valuable insights from this book.

What makes this book all the more remarkable is how it takes a complex subject and translates it into language that is concise and understandable. The content of the book is easy to grasp, yet Dr. Grobstein doesn't talk down to the reader, making this a refreshing guide for anyone seeking the latest knowledge about breast cancer.

The major underlying premise is that patients who have breast cancer must take charge of the critical decisions that will affect their lives. No one else can make these choices, no matter how experienced or well intentioned they may be. Doctors and loved ones can only offer advice, be it based on years of knowledge or on heartfelt emotion. It is the patient who must live with the results.

This message of empowerment reflects the very spirit of the author who has provided quality cancer treatment to breast cancer patients all over the world. Who is this remarkable woman, Dr. Ruth Grobstein? I had the privilege of meeting her at an annual conference of the American Association for Cancer Research almost two decades ago. Taken by her dynamic personality and her strong presence, I was inspired to find out more about her accomplishments as a physician and scientist, along with her perspectives on cancer.

What I discovered was a pioneering woman, one of the world's foremost authorities in radiation oncology, who has dedicated herself to helping cancer patients and saving lives. Married with three children at the age of twenty-eight, she enrolled in a Ph.D. program at Yale University to study developmental biology. At that time, her gender and age set her apart from most of her classmates. In those days, women—particularly married women with children—typically did not go to graduate school.

She followed her vigorous coursework with an even more challenging position as a postdoctoral fellow in biochemistry and pharmacology, and subsequently joined the faculty at the Yale School of Medicine in the department of microbiology. Her research talents were soon recognized. In 1966, she received two major research grants—one from the Atomic Energy Commission and one from the National Institutes of Health—to conduct studies in immunology. That year, she switched coasts to join the faculty at the University of California, San Diego, where she met her now late husband, Clifford Grobstein, Ph.D., a renowned scientist and then chair of the biology department at UCSD, who would become dean of the School of Medicine and a member of the National Academy of Sciences. With the loving support of her husband and a strong desire to make her own mark in the field, she became a highly respected independent contributor to cancer science and medicine. She continues to be a role model for women physicians and scientists everywhere.

During Dr. Grobstein's appointment at UCSD, she decided she wanted to get a medical degree to make a difference in the clinic, so she enrolled at the University of California, Los Angeles. After obtaining her M.D. degree at UCLA, she entered a residency program in radiation oncology. Following the extraordinary tutelage of Dr. Samuel Hellman, a leader in the treatment of breast cancer without mastectomy and an individual who would become a lifelong colleague and friend, she joined the radiation oncology department of the University of California, San Francisco, and established a multidisciplinary clinic that advanced the treatment of breast cancer with lumpectomy rather than mastectomy. Indeed, in San Diego County she was responsible for the shift in the successful treatment of early-stage breast cancer from mastectomy to breast preservation.

Subsequently, Dr. Grobstein became the founder and director of the Ida M. and Cecil H. Green Women's Cancer Program and head of Radiation Oncology at the Scripps Clinic in La Jolla, California. There she combined her years as a bench scientist with her substantive experience as a caring, expert physician.

Throughout her career, Dr. Grobstein never forgot that each patient is an individual and that no two patients' personal lives or medical histories are exactly alike. This is a philosophy she brings to this book, emphasizing time and again that no patient is a statistic and that each person's story is unique. She has listened to the problems of her patients and has responded to their needs.

As its title suggests, Dr. Grobstein's book serves as a personal guide through the myriad questions and decisions that a patient will face in the weeks, months, and years following initial diagnosis. Among other things, her book includes basic definitions of terms, a historical perspective on breast cancer treatment, and diagrams for breast self-examination. It also addresses many of the scientific and medical issues regarding mammography, including what constitutes a "good" mammogram.

There is another unique aspect of the book that the reader will certainly appreciate. The various choices a patient faces when entering the complex world of clinical oncology are organized into decision paths, or "trees," which appear both at appropriate places in the book and gathered at the end, on perforated pages for readers to tear out for easy reference. Dr. Grobstein's goal is to help the patient discover the elements of treatment available at each step along the way. The first decision tree, for example, guides the patient through the initial decisions after a lump is felt or something unusual is seen in a routine mammogram. "What should you do now?" Dr. Grobstein asks. "Look at Decision Tree IA. There are a lot of options. Don't be intimidated; get mobilized, not just because you need to find out if you have breast cancer, but because the combination of uncertainty and inaction will really unsettle you."

The book also serves as a primer on the latest advances in screening technology, treatment options, and research. If breast cancer is diagnosed, the patient is faced with several options, including surgery, chemotherapy, radiation therapy, and some of the newer biological treatments that target tumors without harming surrounding tissue. Because estrogen plays a critical role in the development of hormone-dependent breast cancer, for example, scientists are investigating the therapeutic potential of inhibitors that target the enzymes responsible for stimulating estrogen production in the breast. Other researchers are exploring ways to lessen the side effects of treatment, such as postoperative swelling and pain, to improve the quality of patients' lives. Again, Dr. Grobstein implores the patient to ask questions and to stay in control of decisions that will affect treatment outcome. She encourages readers to question members of the treatment team about their own experience and credentials, and to seek out second and even third opinions when there are differences of opinion. "When a diagnosis of cancer is involved, never fear that you will hurt the feelings of any of your doctors if you ask for a second opinion," she writes. "Competent physicians will never object, as long as the second opinion is obtained from a reputable physician (or group of physicians)." It is this type of advice that gives patients the courage to take charge of their own medical care.

The Breast Cancer Book is an essential resource for anyone who seeks to learn more about breast cancer and how to maximize opportunities for survival. We owe a great debt of gratitude to Dr. Grobstein for giving us the benefit of her extraordinary knowledge and experience in this field.

Margaret Foti, Ph.D., M.D. (h.c.)
Chief Executive Officer
American Association for Cancer Research

Preface

Whether they worry that they might be diagnosed with breast cancer or already have been, women have many reasonable questions about the disease. But they may not allow themselves to ask those questions. This reluctance applies not just to women but to their families and loved ones.

In these days of managed care, patients often are not given enough opportunity to ask questions because the time with their physicians is limited. Patients feel frustrated, hopeless, and angry with their doctors, nurses, schedulers—with a health care system they can't control and with their inability to get answers. They search the Internet and print out a morass of information—but they don't know which bit is useful and which is meaningless. Their frustration grows.

This book is meant not to replace your physicians but to help you get the care you need. It contains simple, straightforward information to enable you to make valid decisions for yourself. Like a trusted friend, it is available to help with some, if not all, of the answers to your questions.

You will find several aids in this book. First are the flow diagrams, or decision trees—a shortcut to help you find the way to appropriate decisions. Think of each decision tree as a map guiding you down a path of decision making, a path that has been followed by other women facing the same kind of problem as you, a path approved by experts in the field of breast cancer.

The text and the decision trees go hand in hand. The text both explains the flow diagrams and gives details needed to make an informed decision. Once you have read the text, you can refer to the decision trees alone when you are thinking through your choices.

Another aid appears at the end of each chapter. It is a series of bulleted points headed "Remember . . . ," which quickly summarizes what you should have learned from the chapter.

The volume is designed so that you need not read it sequentially. You can peruse only the section that concerns you, even if it is midway in the text. The bulleted points and decision trees of preceding chapters may be all you need to get a sense of background. In addition, the decision trees appear again at the end of the book, behind the index, on perforated paper so that you can tear them out for easy reference.

Although I have attempted to keep the book up to date, research in the field is ongoing, and some of the information in this book may not be current at the time you read it. Nevertheless, the general principles are there. This book is a guide, not a tome attempting to tell you all there is to know about breast health or breast cancer. It will give you information to help you make decisions about complex issues like mammography and hormone replacement therapy; it will not tell you everything about the subject.

Most chapters include boxes that contain additional information or give a bit more detail about issues touched on in the text. You don't have to read the boxes in order to understand the text. Think of them as interesting asides, with information you can absorb or set aside. You'll also find figures and diagrams at key points in the discussion. They are meant to facilitate an understanding of the text, so don't skip over them.

This book is intended to simplify your life by giving you enough information to assist you in making wise decisions. I hope it makes the process less of an ordeal.

Acknowledgments

For their sustenance in the writing of this book, I acknowledge the support and loving-kindness of the four persons most important to me: Cliff, Sandy, Beth (Betsy), and Robin. To Jim, Marc, and Abe I say thanks. Nothing would have gone well had it not been for this group of seven.

Fourth daughter Cathy has followed in my footsteps, doing much better than I each step of the way. Her advice and suggestions have been invaluable; most were incorporated into these pages.

Others have been of major assistance in the development of this book. Larry Case, Jonathan Dolger, Jane Isay, and Alida Brill Scheuer never faltered, even when I did. I am immensely grateful to them. My special friends Hinda Rosenthal-Rosenberg and Gloria Schaffer kindly put up with me as house guest during those many visits to Yale University Press.

A number of individuals helped me slog through the difficulties of producing a book. In particular, Jean Thomson Black, Joan Benham, Molly Egland, Tina Weiner, Jenya Weinreb, Nancy Moore, Vivian Wheeler, and Laura Davulis made my life far easier than I had reason to hope. I can never adequately express my gratitude.

The list of resources found at the end of this book was developed at Yale University Press by Kaity Cheng, Laura Davulis, and Nancy Moore.

Finally, I thank the many persons I now regard as friends—those who truly made this book a reality. Several physician specialists were kind enough to read the manuscript, checking for accuracy—Dr. Vivian Lim, Dr. Joan Bull, and Dr. Catherine Park. Friends who have had breast cancer evaluated its relevance to those for whom the book was written. While many others were actively involved in the publication of this book, space is inadequate to cite all the names. I am grateful to each and every one.

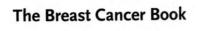

The Breast Cancer Book

Chapter 1   Facts You Should Know and Questions You Might Ask

Are you terrified by the notion that you might have breast cancer? For most women, fear of breast cancer is greater than fear of heart disease, colon cancer, and other cancers. Why this is so is unclear. But women in other Western countries are as frightened of breast cancer as American women. Is it the loss of a breast? Perhaps. In Western countries, breasts are important to a woman's body image. Certainly, fear of breast cancer is greater in developed countries than in developing nations. Western clothing styles can cover up a colostomy. They can even conceal the fact that we have heart disease. But try hiding breasts.

Whether you have been diagnosed with breast cancer or are facing that possibility, do not panic. It may be hard to believe, but you have time. Learn as much about your case as you can before you make a decision about your treatment (Box 1).

Yes, breast cancer is a serious problem and the incidence has been rising. In the United States breast cancer vies with lung cancer as the

---

Box 1 What Is Cancer?

A tumor is an abnormal collection of cells. It can be benign or malignant. Benign tumors—for example, uterine fibroids—can grow to a very large size. But they never metastasize, and their growth is subject to a variety of checks and balances.

"Cancer" refers to a malignant tumor. Cancer cells have two properties that set them apart from benign tumors: (1) they have no control over their growth and can become huge, and (2) they metastasize. That is, cancer cells can enter the blood-stream and be carried to other, more compatible sites in the body, where they can grow without restraint.

Premenopausal women often have breast cancers that are more aggressive-looking under the microscope than those of postmenopausal women. We say they have a higher-grade breast cancer, say grade 2–3 out of a total of three grades $(G\ ^{2-3}/_3)$. It is assumed that high-grade cancers have a shorter doubling time than low-grade cancers. Even if you are pre-menopausal, however, the doubling time still is not so short that you are required to make quick, potentially rash decisions.

---

leading cancer cause of death among women. In recent years lung cancer has won the race (the grim price women have paid for the acceptance of cigarette smoking). First or second, breast cancer is a leading problem for American women. In 2003 there were approximately 211,300 new cases of *invasive* breast cancer plus about 55,700 new cases of *noninvasive* breast cancer. You undoubtedly worry that you may become one of these statistics—if you aren't already.

Here's another statistic, one you may already know. Currently, the lifetime incidence of breast cancer is considered to be one woman in seven. Do you know what this means? If seven 40-year-old women are sitting in a room, do you believe that one of them has (or has had) breast cancer? If you believe that, you are wrong. What one in seven means is that if seven women live to their expected 80+ years, one of them will be diagnosed with breast cancer *during the course of her lifetime.* So if seven 94-year-old women are sitting together in a room, one of them will probably have had a diagnosis of breast cancer. One in seven, like other statistics, has a different significance depending on its context—which, in this instance, is age.

In 1980 the lifetime incidence of breast cancer was regarded to be one woman in eleven. Has a breast cancer epidemic developed in the last twenty-five years? Or does the lifetime incidence of breast cancer appear to be increasing because American women are living longer? The latter undoubtedly comes closer to the truth, although there are many other contributing factors—among them improved mammography, which can diagnose noninvasive and invasive breast cancers even before a lump in the breast is found.

These numbers certainly indicate the magnitude of the breast cancer problem. Now for some numbers that show why you have time to make decisions. How long do you think it takes for one breast cancer cell to divide into two, two into four, four into eight, and so on? Twenty minutes? Twenty-four hours? A few days? A few months? Most people answer twenty minutes or twenty-four hours or even a few days. The correct answer is actually on the order of three months.

A small, pea-sized cancer (one cubic centimeter, the size easily seen on mammograms) is composed of approximately a billion cells. Mathematicians have calculated that it takes thirty doublings to make one billion (that is, to go from one cell to two, to four, to eight, eventually to one billion). You do the arithmetic. Multiply thirty doublings by three months (the time it takes one breast cancer cell to double into two) and you get the astounding number of ninety months, or approximately eight years!

What does this mean for you? It means that if you find a small lump in your breast that turns out to be cancer—even invasive cancer —*and if you are postmenopausal* (older than 50 years), that cancer has been around for a very long time.

What if you are premenopausal? You, too, have time. The dramatic, heartrending scenes in old movies and novels in which a woman with a breast lump is whisked off to the operating room not knowing whether she will emerge with one breast or two—those scenes are gone forever (Box 2).

If you are diagnosed to have breast cancer, two teams will be involved in your care: (1) the diagnostic team, which consists of a radiologist/mammographer, a surgeon (preferably a breast surgeon), and a pathologist; and (2) the treatment team, which comprises a breast surgeon, a radiation oncologist (a specialist who treats cancer with radiation), and a medical oncologist (a specialist who treats cancer with drugs).

When your life is in so many other people's hands, you may feel overwhelmed and passively accept whatever is said to you. Or you may be so confused by the multitude of recommendations that you go into a frenzy and are unable to think straight. You need to keep your wits about you.

Hurried, rash decisions, or decisions made for you by others and accepted by default, will have an impact on the rest of your life. *If you get nothing else from this book, know that you should take the time to explore your options, discuss them thoroughly, and make the right decision for you.* Your decision may not be right (or convenient) for your advisors. But it is yours to make, not theirs.

Well-meaning loved ones and friends may find it easy to give you

Box 2 Breast Cancer—A Brief Historical Perspective

After Wilhelm Conrad Roentgen discovered x-rays at the end of the nineteenth century, radiation was shown to be effective in treating breast cancer. At about the same time, William Steward Halstead, a surgeon, published his first paper on the radical mastectomy. Even though Halstead carried out drastic surgical procedures on women with advanced breast cancer in an era without antibiotics, enough women survived that the Halstead radical mastectomy continued to be the standard of care until the late 1970s.

A consensus meeting of the National Institutes of Health (NIH) in 1979 determined that since rates of survival and recurrence were essentially the same for the radical mastectomy and the modified radical mastectomy, the modified version was preferable. A modified radical mastectomy is far less disfiguring than a radical mastectomy, and has far fewer negative side effects overall. Soon after the consensus meeting, modified radical mastectomy became the new standard of care.

Although the change was heralded, only eleven years later another NIH consensus meeting determined that breast preservation with lumpectomy and radiation yielded results equivalent to modified radical mastectomy. Another new standard was established: less was indeed better.

The trend continues. Today the conventional axillary dissection is being replaced by the lesser sentinel node biopsy, with a concomitant reduction of side effects. Clinical radiation trials are being established to determine whether limited field

continued

continued

irradiation will be equivalent to whole-breast irradiation. The results will not be known for perhaps ten to fifteen years, but radiation oncologists are still trying to do less. Similarly, medical oncologists have shown that women with cancers smaller than one centimeter—who had, by pathology, no breast cancer cells in the lymph nodes under the arm—do not require systemic therapy. They need *neither* chemotherapy nor hormonal manipulation.

advice, often based on their own experiences or those of others. Just remember, the final decision maker is *you*, the patient—not your physician, not your husband, not your mother or close family members or friends. Get their input if you wish; it may be important or it may be simply another old wives' tale. But in the final analysis, you are the decision maker. You—not your loved ones or your friends—have to go to bed each night and wake up with the results of your decision.

A decision between two *equal* alternatives is a gut decision. It is not necessarily the decision others would make. It has to be right for you, the individual woman. It has to *feel* right.

When I counsel a woman who can't make up her mind between two equal alternatives, I often tell her to go to bed one night thinking that she will undergo one of the two treatments, and the next night go to bed persuaded she will have the other. Then she should ask herself on which day she woke up feeling better.

The other side of taking time to decide is that while you do have time, you don't have all the time in the world. Many women, when first told they have breast cancer, don't want this life-changing event to alter the course of their lives. They say, "But I have so much to do . . ." They are frightened. They think adhering to their usual schedule may make the threat go away. A woman who is frightened of having breast cancer—perhaps because she has had an abnormal mammogram, or because she has felt a new lump in her breast—may try to allay her fears by keeping busy taking care of her children, her husband, her career. Women fall easily into this trap, because they have learned the habit of "taking care of."

It's time now to take care of yourself.

If, instead of addressing the problem, you get busy, you are not taking care of yourself, you are not taking hold—*you are not in control.* These circumstances can lead to unfortunate decisions.

Being in control means saying no to other demands. You need to tell others, "I come first, because if I don't, there won't be anything left of me to take care of you." Your children, your husband, your other loved ones cannot know your dread, cannot understand what you are going through when you worry that you have breast cancer. It's up to you to face your problem and make it your first priority. Start by talking to your primary care physician. You're going to have many questions. You need to ask them, and get answers that satisfy you. Don't settle for less.

Yes, I know that in these days of managed care your physician may seem not to have time to answer questions. In fact, your doctor may cringe when he or she sees your list. You may have to make back-to-back appointments to give you enough time for all your questions plus your examination.

Here are some of the questions you may want to ask your doctor if you haven't been diagnosed to have breast cancer.

- I have a lump in my breast that you too can feel. I'm scared. You have referred me for additional studies. When will you tell me about the results? If you can't give me the results, who will?

- You have recommended certain tests. Who has responsibility for giving me the results? When is the earliest that I will know the result of each test you have ordered? Is it possible to get a copy of my test results? If so, will your office send them to me promptly?
- I have a strong family history of breast cancer. Do I need to be checked more frequently than the average person?
- I feel a breast lump. You don't. What should I do? Do I need a mammogram?
- If both you and I feel the same lump in my breast, what do I do about my birth control pills, my hormone replacement therapy, my diet?

Here are some questions you may have if you've been diagnosed with breast cancer.

- What stage am I in? How long will I live? Shall I tell my family?
- Are we certain of the diagnosis? Who is the pathologist who made the diagnosis? What is his or her track record? Do I need a second opinion?
- How will my treatment be decided? What will it be? Must I have surgery? Will I need either chemotherapy or radiation, or both? When?
- Are several treatment teams available? Why did you select this particular team? What is the background of each physician on the team? May I meet each one separately? If I'm not comfortable with a physician on the team, may I choose a replacement?
- If I phone you and you are seeing your routine patients, how soon will you return my phone call—if it is urgent? if it is routine?
- Since I have breast cancer, should my sisters and my female children be checked? How? When?
- Are there support groups that I should join? That my family should meet?
- What can I do to help myself? It's very important that I have some

control over this illness. Should I eat differently? Should I exercise more?

- You are recommending conventional treatments. Will my insurance cover them?
- What alternative or complementary treatments are available? Is one form of treatment mutually exclusive of another? Will my insurance pay for them?

Check with your insurance agent about coverage for tests and treatments.

It is very important to get information about your particular medical system: your hospital, other facilities that may be available, the competence of your diagnosing and treating physicians, second opinions, and so on. You may want to ask your doctor about these issues, or you may want to check other sources. How capable is the radiology department that will be responsible for your mammograms? The pathology department that is responsible for processing and diagnosing your tissue? How competent are the cancer doctors taking care of you? What about the hospital? Is there a cancer nurse coordinator, a social worker, or some other person who can assist you in scheduling tests and with hospitalization—in other words, help you through the system? If you live in a big city, you may have more choices than if you live in a small town.

Set a date for making a decision. Two to four weeks is usually about right. Use the time wisely. And good luck!

Remember . . .
- The pea-sized lump found in your breast or the small density seen in your mammogram probably has been there, undetected, for a very long time. If it is breast cancer, it is not dividing every few minutes or hours or even days. Don't let fear paralyze you—see your physician.

- If you are diagnosed with breast cancer, you have time. Use it wisely. Get as much information as you can about *your* particular breast cancer before you make decisions relating to how it is to be treated.
- When you've received a diagnosis of cancer, no question is too trivial. All questions should be answered promptly.
- If you are postmenopausal, the doubling time for breast cancer generally is on the order of three months. If you are premenopausal, the doubling time may be shorter than that, but you still have time to make decisions based on fact, not fear.
- Set yourself a time limit for decision making. Two to four weeks after the date of your diagnosis is appropriate.
- Be in control of your life. Learn how to handle your breast cancer in the way that suits you best.
- You, and only you, are the final decision maker.

Chapter 2   Detection: Mammograms and Breast Exams

This long chapter has two separate decision trees, Decision Trees 1 and 2. Because of its size, Decision Tree 1 is divided into Decision Tree 1A and Decision Tree 1B. Decision Tree 1A is the path to follow if you have a new breast lump or abnormality. Decision Tree 1B is the path to follow if you haven't. Almost everyone should follow Decision Tree 1B. Essentially, it is a component of breast cancer screening that should be a regular part of your life. Since Decision Tree 1A requires immediate action, we'll start with that.

You may have been examining your breasts since you were in your teens. You know how they normally look and feel. Your doctor probably examines your breasts every year and, depending on your age, you may be getting yearly screening mammograms.

Now there's a lump in your breast that you hadn't noticed before. You discovered it yourself, or your partner did. You have been frantic with anxiety ever since.

Perhaps you're at your doctor's office when the discovery is made.

Decision Tree 1A How to Proceed If You Find a New Lump
in Your Breast

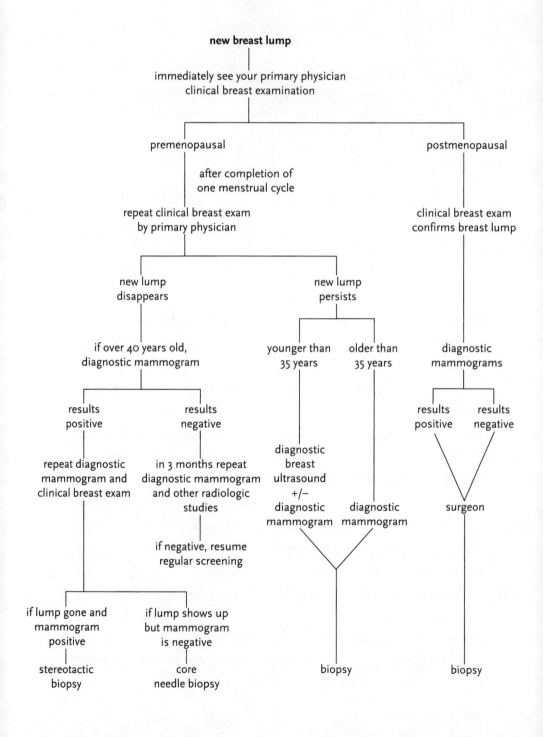

Decision Tree 1B How to Proceed If You Don't Find a New Breast Lump
(Regular Breast Screening)

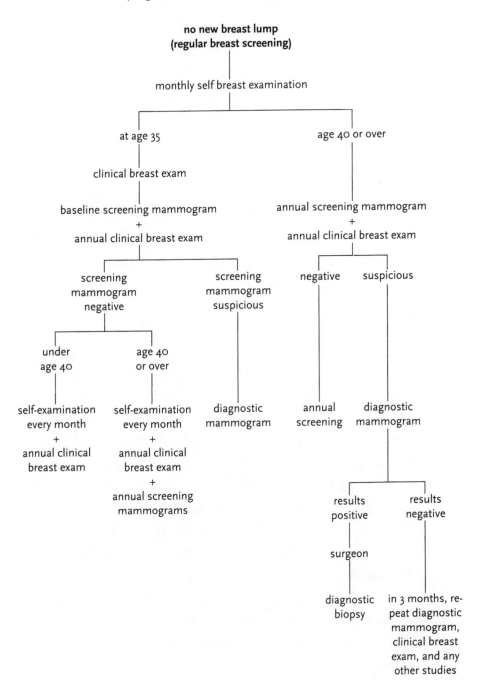

Decision Tree 2 When Your Screening Mammogram
Is Suspicious

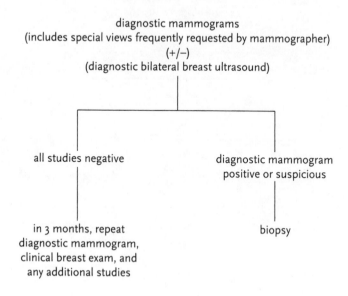

diagnostic mammograms
(includes special views frequently requested by mammographer)
(+/−)
(diagnostic bilateral breast ultrasound)

all studies negative

diagnostic mammogram
positive or suspicious

in 3 months, repeat
diagnostic mammogram,
clinical breast exam, and
any additional studies

biopsy

Your doctor finds a lump during your annual checkup, or the mammographer sees an unusual area in your routine screening mammogram.

What should you do now? Look at Decision Tree IA. There are a lot of options. Don't be intimidated; get mobilized, not just because you need to find out if you have breast cancer, but because the combination of uncertainty and inaction will really unsettle you.

If you haven't already seen your primary physician, do so as soon as possible. He or she can confirm a lump by a clinical breast exam (CBE). Your doctor may not feel a lump even though you do, or even though your mammogram was suspicious. We'll deal with those scenarios later. For now, let's say your doctor confirms the lump you feel. If you are premenopausal, you will be asked to come back within one week of the completion of your next menstrual cycle to ensure that the lump is not a cyst. A painful lump is usually, but not always, a cyst. If you are postmenopausal, you should be sent directly to a surgeon for a biopsy and probably for a mammogram.

Let's say that in a month, or within a week of completion of your next menstrual cycle, neither your self-exam nor your primary physician's exam detects the lump. If you are younger than 35, you may be referred for a diagnostic ultrasound, which can detect cysts and doesn't subject a young woman with radiosensitive breast tissue to radiation.

If you are 35 years old or older, you will be referred for a diagnostic mammogram of both breasts. (The lumpless breast may give information as well.) You will also be sent for a diagnostic mammogram if you had a positive or suspicious screening mammogram but no palpable lump, or if you can feel a lump that your doctor cannot.

If the diagnostic mammogram is positive—that is, it shows a lesion in the breast that had the lump or other abnormality—another diagnostic mammogram and CBE will be performed just to confirm the previous findings. The mammogram could show a lesion that neither you nor your doctor can feel. Or a lump that had gone away could come back, without the diagnostic mammogram's showing any abnormality in the area of the lump. When physical exams and mammograms are at odds, only a biopsy can resolve the issue.

What if the diagnostic mammogram is negative, and neither you nor your doctor can feel or see the lump or abnormality any longer? Is the coast clear? Not quite. As Decision Tree 2 shows, in three months you should (1) repeat the diagnostic mammogram, (2) repeat the CBE, and (3) repeat any other studies, such as breast ultrasound exams.

And then you can resume regular screening for breast cancer.

What if the abnormality doesn't go away after being confirmed by your primary physician's CBE? You too may be referred for a diagnostic mammogram. The bottom line, as in the preceding scenarios, is that you will be sent to have the lesion biopsied. (You'll read about biopsies in Chapter 3.)

Routine Screening for Breast Cancer

Are you confused about how to screen yourself for breast cancer? Certainly the media don't help matters. Conflicting medical issues receive dazzling press attention. Any controversy regarding breast cancer that is found in the medical literature gets reviewed and re-reviewed in the media—frequently before physicians have seen the article cited. The media get the medical journals first, even before the subscribing physicians. As a result of this media coverage, women are seriously confused about how to screen for breast cancer. Many women won't go for mammograms or perform self breast exams (SBEs) or get clinical breast exams (CBEs) from professionals. Some wonder whether radiation from the mammograms will *cause* breast cancer, whether SBEs and/or CBEs are worthless, and whether their physician, who may advocate annual mammograms, is incorrect and old-fashioned. Perhaps even you sometimes ask yourself whether you should believe your doctor, and you wonder where else to turn for accurate, current medical advice. The debate over screening practices isn't likely to end anytime soon, but that's no reason to neglect yourself.

I'll tell you what some of the controversies are. But first I'm going to give you my own advice about screening. Then I'll help you think your way through the maze.

Routine screening of breasts without abnormalities should start with monthly breast exams of yourself beginning at approximately age 18. You'll see from Decision Tree 1B that I recommend a baseline mammogram at 35 years as well as *annual* screening mammograms beginning at age 40. In addition, I recommend a clinical breast exam each year by a qualified physician beginning at any age but no later than 35 years. Let's look at these practices one at a time.

One can argue that SBEs should start when the breasts are fully developed—earlier than at 18 years. The exact time when a girl starts to carry out breast exams on herself is not critical. What is important is that she make monthly self breast exams a habit at an age before she could develop breast cancer.

You may have read that statistically there is no survival benefit from performing regular SBEs. But most women do not know how to examine their own breasts properly. Inadequate SBEs can lead to unsatisfactory statistical results. You will learn how a meaningful self breast exam should be carried out. Understanding that procedure will help you understand whether the physician who carries out your clinical breast exam is doing an effective job. Although statistically the probability that a very young woman will get breast cancer is vanishingly small (the youngest person that I have seen with breast cancer was 18 years old), you are not a statistic.

Clinical breast exams for most women begin during annual check-ups in the office of their primary care physician (or obstetrician or gynecologist). Certainly by age 35 such exams should be routine. Even the efficacy of CBEs has been questioned on statistical grounds because some large population-based studies such as those done by the Women's Health Initiative (WHI) have not shown that lives were saved by clinical breast exams. If you believe your doctor is not performing the CBE adequately, find a doctor who is better at it. You'll be able to tell once you've learned how to examine your own breasts correctly.

Thirty-five is also the age when a woman should have a baseline screening mammogram. You should have your baseline mammogram when you are even younger if you have any breast abnormalities such as multiple cysts, or genetic risk factors such as a strong family history. We call this mammogram a baseline mammogram because your other mammograms will be compared to it.

Baseline mammograms have been questioned because at age 35 a woman's breasts are very dense. Some mammographers feel that it is hard to read young breasts accurately because of the difficulty of assessing abnormalities through the whitish density of the breasts. Still, when done with proper technique (Figure 1), baseline mammograms can detect abnormalities. I feel they are useful and continue to recom-

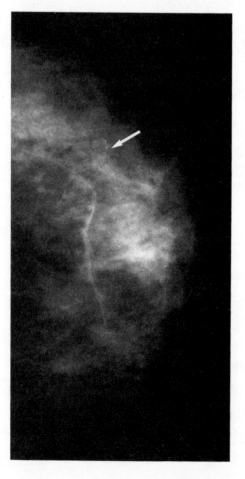

Figure 1 Screening mammogram of a 41-year-old woman. Note that her cancer can be seen (*arrow*) despite a background of dense breast. This woman has a suspicious screening left mammogram; she was asked to return for diagnostic magnification views of the abnormality, which confirmed the lesion.

mend them. If the baseline mammogram shows nothing suspicious, you should continue to screen with monthly examinations of your own breasts and annual CBEs.

From age 40 on, the annual CBE should be done in tandem with an annual screening mammogram. I recommend that you and your doctor should not be satisfied to have only a mammogram report. Your doctor should examine you with the *mammogram itself* in hand to confirm the report. (Note that actual mammograms, which are much larger than the reproductions that appear in this book, must be evaluated by a trained professional.) I urge you to get and keep copies of all your mammograms and other reports.

Until the age of 40, your own examination of your breasts is your most important screening tool. Knowing how to carry out a competent SBE educates you to evaluate the exams your physician performs. It should be a habit you maintain throughout your lifetime.

How to Perform a Self Breast Exam

Start by standing up and looking in the mirror with your hands pressed hard against your hips (Figure 2A). Then put your hands above your head (Figure 2B). In each position, look at your breasts and examine them for symmetry, discoloration, changes in skin texture, warmth, skin "dimpling" or indentations associated with skin creases, redness. Then look at your nipple. Are there any changes such as nipple inversion, scaling, pinkness or redness? Has a nipple been itching?

Then lie down (Figure 2C). *Do not examine your breasts standing up in a shower and/or in a rotary fashion*—you can't be sure you are examining the entire breast. Use either wet, soapy fingers or oil on your fingers to examine your breasts. Even the tinest lump or bump can be detected with slippery fingers. Begin at the center edge of your collar bone (clavicle) just above your breast bone and, pressing deeply, move your four fingers (thumb excluded) back and forth (almost as if you

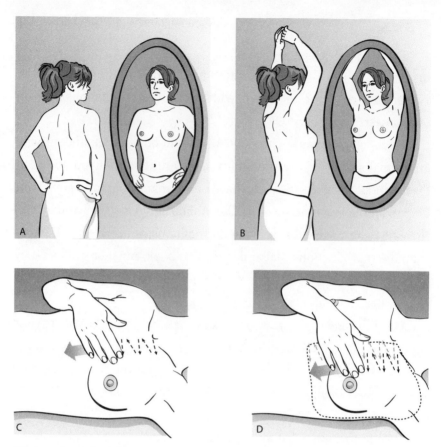

Figure 2 Procedure for carrying out a monthly examination of your breasts, as detailed in text. *A,* Look at yourself in the mirror, placing your hands on your hips. Observe whether either of your breasts is larger or smaller than the other one. Note any redness, swelling, or variation in the texture of your skin. Look at your nipple: Has it changed since your last exam? Is it pink or red, is it scaly, does it itch, is it inverted? Next, press your hands against your hips. Does one breast now have a "dimple"? *B,* Still looking in the mirror, raise your hands above your head straight upward. Do you see a dimple now? Are there changes in either or both breasts? *C,* Now lie down. Examine your breasts in a linear (not circular) fashion. *D,* Your four borders are: (1) upper border: medial edge of your collar bone (clavicle), which is on top of your breast bone (sternum); (2) medial border: down from the upper border, 1–2 inches toward the other breast to 2–3 inches below your breast crease; (3) lower border: 2–3 inches below your breast crease; (4) lateral border: 2–3 inches below the breast toward the underarm. Begin your exam at the upper medial border. With the flat of the four fingers on your opposite hand, examine your breast in a linear strip until you reach the lower border. Overlap each strip that you examine so that no part of your breast is unexamined. When through, squeeze and look at your nipple to be sure there is no discharge or change. Once you have examined your breasts, examine your armpits as described in the text.

were having long, sustained shudders), going down the entire length of your breast to approximately three inches below the lowest part of your breast.

When you have completed examining this first strip of breast tissue, overlap the first strip and use the same technique to go down the adjacent strip of your breast. Continue in this fashion until you have completely covered your breast and have extended beyond it by about two to three inches (Figure 2D).

Next, look at each nipple and squeeze it to see if any fluid comes out. If so, what color is it—red, brown, green? Also note if the nipple is red or pink, scaly, or itchy.

The value of such an exam is that you are using a firm surface, your chest wall, against which to press your breasts. If your breasts are large, pendulous, and floppy, roll yourself around so that you can always examine your breast against your firm chest wall.

When you have completed examining your breast with deep pressure, repeat your exam using gentle pressure. Your breast will feel entirely different during the two exams.

The texture of a normal breast is like oatmeal: it is not smooth. Many tiny, normal glands contribute to this texture. A dominant mass is one that stands out from the oatmeal-like background and does not merge with the underlying tissue when you flatten your fingers and rub over the surface of the lump. If you find a dominant mass, note whether it has a smooth, slippery surface or a slightly rough surface. Notice also whether it is mobile or attached to surrounding, contiguous tissue, drawing the overlying skin down and producing an indentation or dimple in the skin.

Now make a diagram of your breasts, being sure that you date your diagram and note where you see and/or feel any abnormalities (Figure 3A). Specify whether you see any changes in your breast of the sort noted in the mirror. You can think of your breast as a clock: twelve

A   date: xx/yy/zzzz

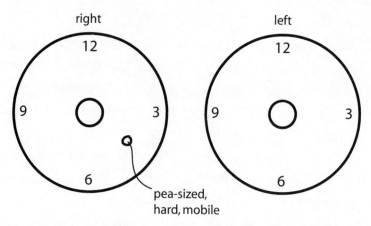

Figure 3A One method of diagramming significant abnormal findings. Think of your breasts as clocks. Indicate abnormalities as breast lumps, giving them a size and a location. Be sure to date your drawing. In this example, you have felt a pea-sized lump at four o'clock in your right breast.

o'clock is at the top/center of each breast, while three o'clock is at the outside of your left breast and on the inside of your right breast. Some common kitchen items are reasonable estimates of size. For example, a garden pea is approximately one centimeter. A pitted olive is about two centimeters. A small egg is three to four centimeters. Note whether any mass that you feel is tender. Again, if you have any nipple changes or discharges, note them. Your diagram will be extremely valuable if you bring it to show the radiologist reading your mammograms, and to your examining physician.

After you have completed the examination of your breasts, turn your attention to the lymph nodes in your armpit—your axilla (Figure 3B). Relax your arm so that the axilla will be soft. Place your four fingers (excluding the thumb) as high in the axilla as you can get. Then sweep downward, pressing against the hard surface of your chest wall as you go. This maneuver will probably require some practice. You may

B   date: xx/yy/zzzz

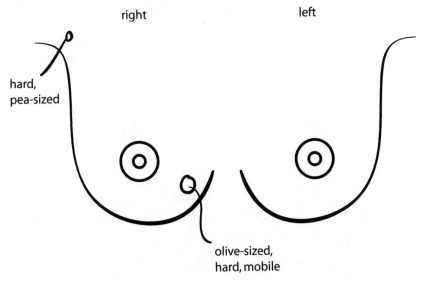

Figure 3B This alternative diagram encourages you to remember the lymph nodes in your armpit. Here you have an olive-sized, hard, mobile lump at four o'clock in your right breast and a hard, pea-sized mass in your right axilla.

have to perform it repeatedly to check for any firm, pea-sized structure in your axilla.

Inflammatory Breast Cancer

You should know the symptoms of inflammatory breast cancer— not because it is so prevalent, but because it is so dangerous. If it is not treated appropriately, inflammatory breast cancer can become a major disaster.

In the past, inflammatory breast cancer has been a clinical diagnosis. That is, a trio of characteristics in the physical exam led one to say, "This is inflammatory breast cancer." If all three findings were not present *at one time*, it was probably not inflammatory breast cancer. The three characteristic breast findings are redness, warmth, and a *peau d'orange* appearance of the skin of the breast. Also—and this is important—a very large breast mass can always be found in association with the three characteristic breast changes.

A few words about the trio of breast skin changes. The so-called redness of the breast skin is not generally red. It ranges from a reddish color to pink, like a flush. It does not necessarily cover the entire breast; it can merely cover one part of the breast. It can be very subtle.

The redness is associated with warmth. That is, the area of the breast that is pink or red is also warm. You can easily feel the warmth with your hand, as if you were feeling the feverish forehead of a child.

The third change associated with the pink-to-red warm skin of the breast is peau d'orange; the skin of the breast has the texture of the skin of an orange, being thick and lightly pitted. It is often the first sign that one is dealing with inflammatory breast cancer. It results from edema (fluid) in the skin. The other changes may be very subtle and noticed only after finding peau d'orange.

I add another feature: a very large, central breast mass. Although the mammogram report may be negative, when serial mammograms are examined closely, invariably a poorly defined, large central density is seen. If the breast is then carefully palpated, a large, central mass that fills almost the entire breast is found. If inflammatory breast cancer is suspected, be sure to have a biopsy. Pathologic changes, such as cancer cells in the lymph ducts in the skin (dermal lymphatics), are characteristic of inflammatory breast cancer.

Mammography

By age 35 you should have had your first screening mammogram, and after age 40 you should have one every year. This recommendation is still controversial, but I make it without hesitation. In a moment I'll explain why.

But first, you may be wondering how screening mammograms are different from the diagnostic mammograms you've read about here or elsewhere. *Screening mammograms* are just that; they screen apparently normal breasts for breast cancer. Two standard views are taken of the right breast and two of the left breast—a total of four views per patient. One view is taken from above, the so-called cradio-caudal view; the other is taken from the side, the lateral view. In each view, it is important to visualize the entire breast.

Decision Tree 2 shows you what to do if your screening mammogram shows a suspicious area (for example, a density that could be cancer, or tiny "clustered" calcifications). The radiologist or mammographer reading your screening mammogram may recommend a *diagnostic mammogram* (see Figure 4). Usually, a diagnostic mammogram consists of a one-sided (right or left) mammogram taken with special views to enable the mammographer to determine whether the abnormality that was seen on the screening film is suspicious enough to warrant a biopsy. The mammographer reading the screening mammogram often will indicate what additional studies should be done to further evaluate the screening abnormality.

Being asked to return for additional studies doesn't mean that you have breast cancer. It means that your mammographer is being very careful. *Most repeat mammograms reveal no cancer.* Read that sentence twice because it is important to remember. If you are called back to have a diagnostic mammogram, don't panic. Additional studies are often ordered simply to clarify your screening mammogram—for example, if the entire breast was not visualized in one or both views. Or a subtle new density that was seen may in fact be the result of a "confluence of shadows." Repositioning you and repeating the mammogram may eliminate the problem.

If, however, your radiologist wishes to follow a suspicious density or microcalcifications in your breast, he or she may recommend re-

A

Left   **Right**

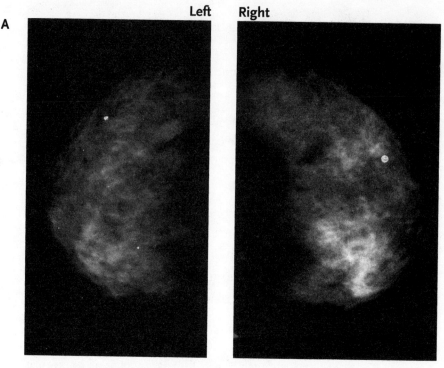

Figure 4A Mammogram showing coarse, benign calcifications scattered in the right breast and one large, benign calcification in the left breast.

peating the diagnostic study in six months. That could be too long to wait if the abnormality turns out to be cancer, especially if you are premenopausal. I recommend an interval of three months for a repeat diagnostic mammogram as well as for the recommended studies plus a thorough clinical breast exam.

Do not shorten the three-month interval between mammograms. If you do, no change may be detected and the unchanged mammogram will convey a false sense of security. Even three months may be too short an interval to show change. That is why, if there is no change, I recommend *two* repeat mammograms—one at three months, the second three months later (at six months). Then, if your radiologist feels there is little likelihood that you have cancer, he or she will recom-

Left

B

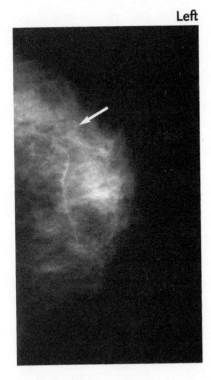

Figure 4B Suspicious, clustered microcalcifications in the screening mammogram of the left breast.

mend returning to annual screening mammograms. If the density seen in your mammogram remains suspicious, a biopsy should be carried out.

Let me repeat: *Always ask for a copy of your mammogram report.* In fact, you should keep a complete file of all your studies, whether they are mammogram reports or operation reports or pathology reports. If your health care is not in a single institution that keeps individual patient charts, you may be the only person to have a complete set of reports covering your health care immediately available.

A recent media storm has raged concerning the value of screening mammograms. The controversy stemmed from an article by two Belgian researchers, published in the respected journal *The Lancet* on October 20, 2001. It criticized studies carried out over the previous thirty years, which showed that screening mammography saved the lives of up to 30 percent of the women screened. Early detection had caught their cancers at an early, potentially curable stage. Five-year studies, even ten-year studies, are frequently not long enough; breast cancer is an indolent disease. The conclusions of the thirty-year studies formed the basis of the National Cancer Institute (NCI) and the American Cancer Society (ACS) recommendations, which favored regular screening mammograms beginning at age 40.

The two Belgian researchers claimed that the long-term studies were flawed on procedural and statistical grounds and therefore had reached invalid conclusions. Their article caused a sensation both in the lay press and in medical and scientific journals. Medical researchers, after evaluating the Belgian study and performing their own statistical analyses, came to a variety of conclusions. A few confirmed and most negated the Belgian study. The press, instead of addressing the procedural and statistical issues that had been raised, had a field day. Many women, reading the sensational press releases, became so confused that they doubted they would get mammograms—ever.

The bottom line for you is that, regardless of the flaws cited by critics of the thirty-year study, *screening mammograms saved lives.* The NCI and ACS reaffirmed their recommendation of screening mammograms despite the furor over the *Lancet* article (Box 3). As a result of their recommendations as well as those of other respected cancer agencies, most health insurance companies today will pay for screening mammograms every one or two years for *all* women 40 years of age and older.

If you are 40 to 50 years of age, you are thought erroneously to be in a lower risk category than older women. Most health insurance companies will pay for this 40 to 50 group only every other year and some won't pay for this group at all. But many medical researchers point out that although your statistical risk of being diagnosed with breast cancer is lower, if you *are* diagnosed with breast cancer, the

Box 3 Recommendations on Screening Mammograms

In response to an article published in *The Lancet* of October 20, 2001, which questioned the value of mammography, the following recommendations were issued:

National Cancer Institute Recommendations updated May 3, 2002:

- "Women in their 40s and older should have mammograms every one to two years."
- "Women who are at higher than average risk of breast cancer should talk with their health care providers about whether to have mammograms before age 40 and how often to have them."

U.S. Department of Health and Human Services Recommendations updated February 21, 2002:

- HHS Secretary Tommy Thompson announced an updated recommendation from the U.S. Preventive Services Task Force (USPSTF) that calls for "screening mammography, with or without clinical breast examination, every one to two years for women ages 40 and over. This recommendation affirms HHS's existing position on the value of mammography."
- The USPSTF made two earlier breast cancer screening recommendations, in 1989 and 1996, that endorsed mammography for women over 50 years of age.
- The USPSTF acknowledged that some risks were associated with mammography (for example, false positives leading to unnecessary biopsies and surgeries), but noted that these risks lessen as women get older.

breast cancer is likely to be a more aggressive, more dangerous form. With the stakes so high, do you really want to stand by and count on the odds being in your favor?

It is true that some suspicious lesions seen on screening mammograms have been subjected to unnecessary tests. For example, many women with suspicious densities or suspicious microcalcifications on their screening mammograms were found, upon further investigation, to have no cancer. A cost-benefit analysis indicated that it was overly costly to perform screening mammograms—the pickup rate of cancers was too low when compared to the high pickup rate and cost of detecting benign, noncancerous lesions.

Do you want a cost-benefit analysis to apply to your life? What if you were the woman found to have an early-stage, potentially curable breast cancer? Wouldn't you be glad to know this as early as possible, so that you would have a greater chance to preserve your breast without sacrificing a cure (Box 4)?

The issue of radiation and mammograms has been another favorite subject of the press. If you are a woman who won't get a mammogram because of your fear that the radiation involved can cause cancer, here is information for you:

- Radiation is emitted from current mammography equipment in state-of-the-art mammography centers.
- Radiation can cause cancer. Radiation to the breast can cause breast cancer.
- Low-dose radiation to *susceptible* breast tissue can cause breast cancer.
- The total radiation dose can be cumulative. Therefore, multiple exposures of radiation to the same site are additive. If a very low dose of radiation is delivered multiple times to the same site (to the breast), the *total* dose may be cancer inducing, even though the single, very low dose of radiation would not cause cancer.

Box 4 National Cancer Institute Statement on the
Benefits and Limitations of Screening Mammograms
(reviewed May 3, 2002)

Benefits:
- Several worldwide studies have shown that screening mammograms reduced the number of breast cancer deaths in
women aged 40 to 69 years. The reduced mortality was predominantly in the group of women over age 50. In these
studies, no clear-cut benefit was shown for women younger
than 40 years, either from regular screening mammograms
or from baseline screening mammograms.

Limitations:
- If a cancer is detected by screening mammography, it is not
necessarily the case that the affected woman's life will be saved.
Some cancers are very aggressive; even though they may be
tiny or not felt during a physical examination, they may have
spread to other parts of the body by the time they are detected.
- A screening mammogram may be falsely *negative*. In other
words, the mammogram may not show a cancer that is, in
fact, present. In approximately 20 percent of mammograms,
cancers that subsequently develop are not detected.

- *The dose of radiation you receive when you get a mammogram is so low
that it is not cancer causing. When the doses from screening plus diagnostic mammograms over multiple years are added, the total dose does
not come close to the dose needed to cause breast cancer.*

Table 1 Comparative amounts of radiation from various sources

Source of radiation	Approximate annual dose
Natural background radiation in United States*	90 mrem[†]
One transatlantic flight from United States to Europe[‡]	5 mrem
Man-made sources of radiation:	
Medical	
Mammogram (standard to digital)[§]	< 30 mrem
Chest x-ray (2 views)	< 0.5 to 1 mrem
Nonmedical	
Television, computers, and the like	2 mrem
Nuclear power (estimate for year 2000)	< 1 mrem

* Natural background radiation arises from three sources: (1) cosmic rays from outer space; (2) radioactivity from the earth and from buildings; (3) self-exposure from inhaled or ingested radioactive products. Radiation exposure from the natural background totals 90 mrem *annually.*

[†] The rem is a unit of the dose we absorb when we are exposed to radiation. One rem is approximately equal to one rad, which is an amount of radiation delivered from a source of radiation. A millirem (mrem) or millirad is one thousandth of a rem or rad (0.001 rem or rad).

[‡] A person traveling from the United States to Europe absorbs approximately 5 mrem from cosmic radiation. The pilot of a jetliner who makes regular transatlantic flights (on northerly routes) or transcontinental flights absorbs approximately 500 mrem per year—technically rendering this pilot a radiation worker.

[§] A standard screening mammogram (two views of each breast or a total of four views) delivers less radiation to the breast than six transcontinental or transatlantic trips. This dose is not genetically significant and probably will not cause genetic mutations.

Source: Adapted from Eric Hall, *Radiobiology for the Radiologist,* 2nd ed., Harper and Row, 1998, and from G. Mitchell and L. Bassett, Eds., *The Female Breast and Its Disorders,* Williams & Wilkins, 1990.

- Table 1 compares the radiation from mammograms to the radiation received from other sources.
- Your age at the time of your mammograms is a vital factor. I stated above that low-dose radiation to *susceptible* breast tissue can cause breast cancer. Developing breast tissue is susceptible breast tissue; it is found primarily in girls and women between the ages of 13 and 30 years. Women 35 or 40 years of age and older do not have susceptible breast tissue.
- Thus, the two crucial factors contributing to breast cancer from radiation are dose and age.
- False negative mammograms are seen more frequently in young women. These premenopausal women often have dense breasts that make it difficult for the mammographer or radiologist to see through the glandular tissue. In a study I carried out at Scripps Clinic in La Jolla, California, women younger than age 40 had predominantly high-grade (more aggressive) cancers when compared to a group of postmenopausal women older than 50 years. The combination of dense breasts and more aggressive cancers makes premenopausal women very vulnerable.
- The screening mammogram may be falsely *positive*. That is, the radiologist or mammographer may see something "suspicious," which requires additional study. About 80 percent of breast abnormalities seen on mammograms prove not to be cancer at all when studied further.
- A false positive mammogram can be very distressing to a patient who is intensely frightened by the notion that she may have breast cancer. A quick resolution is not necessarily forthcoming (scheduling may be difficult). Imagine her relief when she is told that the density seen on the mammogram is not cancer at all!

   If you are in the age group with susceptible breast tissue—between 13 and 30 years—you should avoid all radiation to your breasts, including mammography. And whatever your age, make sure that *the mammography center where you get your mammograms is* state of the art *and certified by the Food and Drug Administration (FDA)*. If it is, you can be assured that the dose put out by the mammography equipment is far below the dose that can cause breast cancer. Certification by the FDA means, among other things, that the equipment is routinely checked by a qualified radiation physicist. The American College of Radiology (ACR) can also accredit mammography equipment based on FDA guidelines. Look for a certificate of accreditation (which must be prominently displayed) in the center that you choose, regardless of the country in which you have your mammogram (Box 5). Be sure it is up to date. Your life could depend on it.

In addition to being sure that your mammograms are taken in a certified center, be certain that they are read by a radiologist who is an expert in reading mammograms. What is an expert mammographer? In my view, that person should read between 2,500 and 5,000 mammograms per year and make very few errors. In addition, he or she should insist on working with outstanding technologists. An outstanding mammography technologist is one who, among other things, always positions the patient so that the entire breast is included in each of the two views per breast and who insists that all of the patient's prior mammograms are available at the time the current films are read.

In the United Kingdom, where the health care system is regulated by the government, mammographers are required to read 5,000 mammograms per year. As a result, the error rate is very low. In contrast, the United States has set a minimum standard of only 480 mammograms to be read per year by a mammographer. Many radiologists in this country argue that the number is too low and is frequently associated with false negatives—mammograms in which cancers have been missed—as well as false positives. Don't be afraid to ask the average number of mammograms read annually by the person reading

Box 5 Finding an Appropriate Mammography Center

The Mammography Quality Standards Act (MQSA) was designed to ensure that every mammography center will meet
certain standards set by the U.S. government in 1999. Each
mammography department, whether it is hospital based, pri-
vate, or a mobile van, must be certified for adherence to the
standards set by the Food and Drug Administration. Not only
must the equipment meet those criteria, but so too must the
associated personnel. Once all the standards are met, the facility will be issued a certificate, which should be prominently displayed. You will want to check that the expiration date has not
passed.

If these requirements are not met, find a facility where they are.

your mammogram. If it is below 2,500, I recommend you go some-
where else.

You may have heard about breast ultrasound, and you wonder if it
might be a better screening technique for breast cancer since it does
not require radiation. The answer is that breast ultrasound is a satisfactory adjunct to mammography, but it does not replace mammography
—for the following important reason: a breast ultrasound (or breast
echogram) is best used to detect fluid-filled masses. For example, if a
mass is detected on your mammogram, a breast ultrasound may be
recommended because it can readily determine whether the mass is
actually a cyst (generally a benign, fluid-filled lesion). Mammograms
detect cysts but don't readily distinguish them from suspicious solid

masses. In such a case, breast ultrasound is used as a *diagnostic* tool, not a *screening* tool. If the patient having the breast ultrasound is found to have a cyst, a needle attached to a syringe can be visualized going directly into the cyst. The fluid of the cyst can be aspirated (sucked out through the syringe), thereby immediately making the diagnosis as well as alleviating any symptoms of pain from the cyst.

Mammography is the best screening technique we have to date, although other options are on the horizon. Mammographers can grade the level of suspiciousness of a mammogram by using a code in their reports—for example, the ACR code (Box 6).

Box 6 ACR (American College of Radiology) Code

In accordance with the Mammography Quality Standards Act of April 28, 1999, all patients must be informed of their screening mammography results. Based on ACR Code 0, the results from all patients with abnormal findings are to be reported.

American College of Radiology Rating System

ACR 0 = abnormal; requires additional imaging

ACR 1 = negative findings

ACR 2 = benign findings

ACR 3 = six-month follow-up

ACR 4 = suspicious

ACR 5 = very suspicious

Note: Some mammography facilities use the MAFI system rather than the ACR system. A code of MAFI 1 (abnormal result) is the same as ACR 0, and MAFI 0 is equal to ACR 1 or ACR 2.

Mammograms are not perfect. Sometimes they detect too much, sometimes they detect too little. Sometimes (10–15 percent of the time) they do not even detect a lump that was readily felt by you or your physician. Don't rely on a negative mammogram report. Lobular cancers (described in Chapter 4) may not have very distinct borders and are notorious for being associated with negative mammograms. I always say to the medical students and residents I teach, "A lump is cancer unless it is proven otherwise." I say it to you as well. If you or your physician feels a lump in your breast, it is cancer until it is proven otherwise. Only a biopsy will tell the story.

Remember . . .

- Physical exams and mammograms currently are the two ways of screening your breasts for abnormalities that might be cancer.
- Screening mammograms are x-rays of the "normal" breast. They are done on women who have not noted any breast changes and whose physician has not noted any suspicious findings. Diagnostic mammograms are special views of the breast that are taken when screening mammograms show suspicious changes or when a physical examination of the breast indicates an abnormality.
- Have a baseline screening mammogram at age 35. Assuming that no abnormalities are found, have *annual* mammograms starting at age 40 and continuing *each year* for the rest of your life.
- Examine your breasts every month starting at age 18 or earlier. Learning to examine your breasts properly will enable you to judge how well your physician carries out the clinical breast exam.
- CBEs should begin no later than at age 35.
- The unit (the equipment, and personnel including the radiologist, the radiology technologists, and the radiological physicist) responsible for carrying out your mammography should exceed the minimum standards. Look for a certificate stating that the mammogra-

phy unit has fulfilled the necessary criteria to be federally accept-able. Be sure that the certificate is up to date.

• Obtain and keep copies of all your mammography reports. Once you get used to doing this, you won't hesitate to ask for other re-ports you may need.

Chapter 3   The Path to Your Diagnosis:
Breast Biopsies

Your primary care physician has confirmed the lump you feel. It may or may not have shown up on your screening mammogram. Or there's no palpable lump, but a routine mammogram looked suspicious and you've been referred for a diagnostic mammogram.

The mammographer who carries out your diagnostic mammogram is a member of your diagnostic team. The other two members are your pathologist and your surgeon.

Mammographers can grade the level of suspiciousness by using a code in their report—for example, the ACR code (see Box 6, in Chapter 2). But a diagnosis cannot be made until a biopsy is performed and the pathologist looks at the biopsied tissue under the microscope. *Only the pathologist can make the diagnosis.*

Thus, you must have a biopsy if you want to know what the abnormality in your mammogram really is. In most cases, you will need to see a surgeon, preferably one who specializes in breast cancer.

As you look at Decision Tree 3, you'll see that it is divided into two

Decision Tree 3 Breast Biopsies

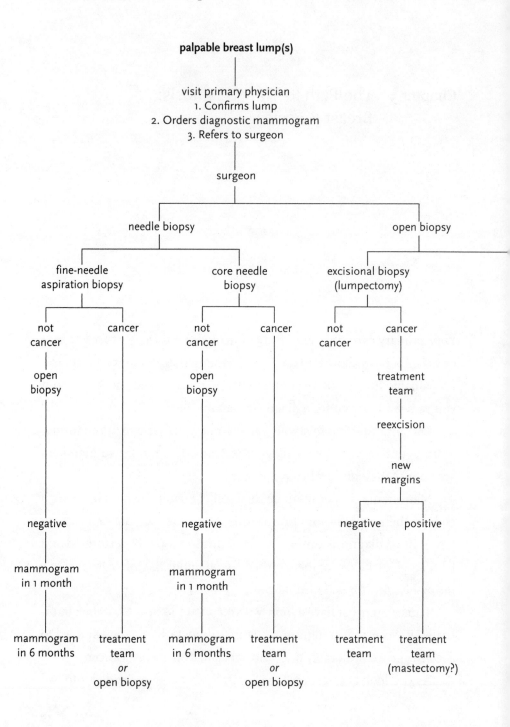

palpable breast lump(s)

visit primary physician
1. Confirms lump
2. Orders diagnostic mammogram
3. Refers to surgeon

surgeon

needle biopsy   open biopsy

fine-needle   core needle   excisional biopsy
aspiration biopsy   biopsy   (lumpectomy)

not   cancer   not   cancer   not   cancer
cancer   cancer   cancer

open   open   treatment
biopsy   biopsy   team

                                                               reexcision

                                                               new
                                                               margins

negative   negative   negative   positive

mammogram   mammogram
in 1 month   in 1 month

mammogram   treatment   mammogram   treatment   treatment   treatment
in 6 months team   in 6 months team   team   team
             or   *or*   (mastectomy?)
             open biopsy   open biopsy

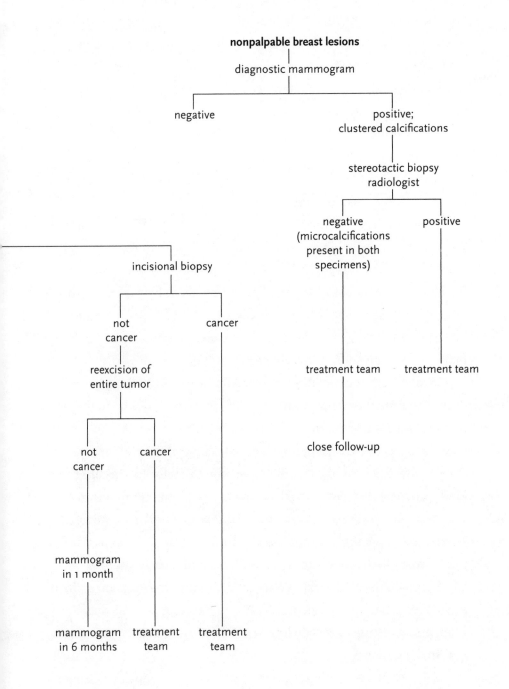

main branches. The one on the left is entitled "palpable breast lump(s)"; the one on the right, "nonpalpable breast lesions." The lump in your breast that you can feel is a "palpable" lump. The "nonpalpable" lesion refers to a lesion you cannot feel, but your mammogram is abnormal. Palpable lumps are more common than nonpalpable lesions, so we'll start with them.

After finding your breast lump, you already have gone to your primary care physician, who simultaneously arranges for you to have a diagnostic mammogram and refers you to a surgeon. The surgeon confirms your breast lump and recommends a biopsy.

Since you have a palpable lesion, it can be biopsied in one of two ways: (1) by a needle biopsy, which is an office procedure, or (2) by an open biopsy, which is carried out in the operating room. A nonpalpable abnormality also can be biopsied by a needle biopsy; this procedure, called a stereotactic biopsy, is carried out by a trained mammographer in a specially equipped radiology suite. I'll explain each of these biopsies in detail later in this chapter.

Far less tissue is involved in a needle biopsy than in an open biopsy. The time the tissue from a needle biopsy needs to be in the initial fluid (known as the fixative) is significantly shorter. As a result, it takes less time for the pathologist to make a diagnosis.

For most people, time is the determining factor in choosing the kind of biopsy. If your primary doctor confirms the lump and refers you to a general surgeon, very likely the surgeon will be unable to schedule an appointment for you right away; a week or so in the future is typical. This delay adds to the stress and anxiety you feel. Mercifully, a core needle biopsy can be carried out in the surgeon's office at your original appointment. There's no waiting for the operating room and the surgeon's schedule to mesh, as would be the case if you had an open biopsy.

Likewise, if a screening mammogram shows a nonpalpable abnormality, a stereotactic biopsy can be scheduled in the radiology suite. The time-limiting factor in this case is coordination of the scheduling of the specially equipped room and the mammographer.

The Needle Biopsy

A needle biopsy can be performed in most circumstances. Let's say you have a palpable lump. Look at the left branch of the decision tree. You can see that there are two types of needle biopsies: a fine-needle aspiration (FNA) and a core needle biopsy. Both are carried out on palpable lumps as office procedures, but the techniques are not the same. In addition, different pathologists are involved: a highly trained cytopathologist reads (and may perform) the FNA, whereas a surgical pathologist reads a core needle biopsy.

The Fine-Needle Aspiration Biopsy

The advantage of an FNA is that it is the quickest way to demonstrate the presence of cancer. If cancer is shown to be present, a definitive diagnosis has been made and days of anguished waiting are eliminated. A positive diagnosis of cancer by an FNA resolves the issue of whether you do or don't have cancer. The drawback is that a negative FNA gives no meaningful information. Because of the way an FNA is carried out, a false negative is possible.

A fine-needle aspiration biopsy is carried out with a small syringe and needle—essentially like the ones used to give you a flu injection or a DPT (diphtheria, pertussis, and tetanus) shot when you were a small child. The syringe and the needle are used to suck out (aspirate) some cells from the lump for an examination under the microscope.

Often, if an unskilled person performs the FNA, no cells appear in the aspirate. The FNA has two requirements: cells must be obtained, and the aspirate must be properly prepared for the cytopathologist to read. In some facilities, the cytopathologist carries out the FNA and also looks at the stained cells under the microscope, thereby giving the patient an answer almost immediately.

If cells from the lump are not present or if the cells are not prepared properly for the pathologist, a diagnosis cannot be made and the report will read "nondiagnostic." A negative FNA doesn't mean anything, for cancer may be present in spite of a negative report. This is what we have called a false negative.

To be certain that there is no cancer, the surgeon needs to carry out an open biopsy, in which the *entire* suspicious area is surgically removed (an excisional biopsy). If a valid excisional biopsy proves to be negative (that is, no cancer is found), you can be assured that you do not have cancer in that particular suspicious area of your breast.

If the FNA diagnosis is positive (cancer is present), each member of the treatment team should be consulted—the breast surgeon, the breast radiation oncologist, and the breast medical oncologist. Even though you think you know whether or not you wish to preserve your breast, you may not have the entire picture. Listen carefully to each specialist before making up your mind how you wish to proceed. In this instance, four heads are better than one.

The Core Needle Biopsy

If a lump is palpable, a core needle biopsy or an FNA can be carried out. If you want to know whether you have cancer, either biopsy will serve—but only if the result is positive.

How is a core needle biopsy different from an FNA? Why does a different pathologist read it? At best, the FNA obtains only cells. A core needle obtains a thin sample of the tissue itself and views all the cells in their proper architectural relation to other cells in the tissue. So the core needle biopsy gives more information than the FNA.

A special cutting needle obtains several thin cores of tissue from the suspicious area, which are then placed in a standard "fixing" solution that prepares the tissue for the pathologist. Because the cores are so thin, the time in the fixing solution is much shorter than the time necessary for the much larger piece of tissue from an open biopsy. Once the tissue is prepared and stained, the pathologist examines it under the microscope and makes a diagnosis.

What will the pathologist say? First, you will be informed whether cancer is or is not present—whether the biopsy is positive or negative. If cancer is present in the core biopsy, the pathologist generally can get enough information from the architecture of the tissue to tell you the type of cancer that you have and also how orderly the cells are (the grade). Pathologists also can give you information about whether the cancer they are seeing has special attributes such as estrogen and/or progesterone receptors, but such information is usually obtained from an open biopsy, where a larger piece of tissue can be obtained.

Be sure you understand that pathologists are limited to what they see. They cannot comment on tissue other than the thin core they are seeing under the microscope. *They diagnose only what they see.*

If the core needle biopsy is positive, cancer is present and your next decision is how you want your breast cancer to be treated.

It is not so easy if the core needle biopsy is negative. You may need an open biopsy to get more information. Consult with all three members of your treatment team. They can explain the issues and guide you.

What if you do not have a palpable lump, but you need a biopsy because you have a suspicious mammogram? As you can see on the right side of the decision tree, a stereotactic biopsy makes it possible to carry out a biopsy on lesions that are not palpable but visible only on a mammogram.

Suppose the screening mammogram shows a cluster of suspicious microcalcifications deep in your breast. Microcalcifications are believed to be formed as a result of cells that have died in the breast duct system. The dead cells and their debris become calcified and are visible as if they were multiple tiny white grains. Calcifications that indicate cancer can be seen either in association with a mass or long before a lump has been detected, as in the example depicted in Figure 4B. The microcalcifications are seen well in the magnification mammogram and, when not associated with a lump, can be effective indicators of noninvasive ductal carcinoma. These calcifications can be sampled by the mammographer in the specially equipped mammography suite, or they can be totally removed by a surgeon in a procedure known as a needle localization biopsy. Regardless, the initial part of the procedure is the same.

You will be taken to the special mammography room and asked to lie, stomach down, on a table that has an opening through which your involved breast will hang. A mammogram will be taken of this breast in position to locate the nonpalpable lesion to be studied. Once the suspicious lesion is seen, a specially designed computer will localize it. The specially trained mammographer will guide a needle into the localized area and, using a needle through which a tiny metal (nontoxic) marker is extruded, place this tiny marker into the localized area. Once the area is localized, a cutting core needle will be inserted into the area; a bit of tissue containing the calcifications will be removed into the cutting core needle. This is the core. Generally, several cores will be taken. These cores will be placed in a fixing fluid and submitted to the pathologist.

The entire procedure takes less than an hour. You can then go home.

If the area with calcifications is to be surgically excised (an open biopsy), the procedure is more complex: it involves both the mammographer and the surgeon plus the operating room and special radiographic equipment. It takes more time. The procedure is known as a stereotactic localization excisional biopsy. The mammographer stereotactically localizes the suspicious lesion (generally with a wire that projects out of the breast), and the surgeon carries out the excisional biopsy. (Details of the procedure are given a little later in this chapter.)

The Open Biopsy

An open biopsy generally is carried out by your breast surgeon in the operating room. It consists of a surgical incision, generally directly above the area to be removed, and removal of some or all of the involved tissue. The surgeon describes his or her findings in an "operation report," which must be dictated and signed by the surgeon after each surgical procedure. Surgical findings can include a description of the tissue as soft, hard, gritty, and the like. Often, the characteristics of the tissue described in the surgical findings suggest cancer.

A surgeon may say "It's cancer" and "I got it all out." Your two burning questions are answered. But what the surgeon *really* means is "It's *probably* cancer" and "I got all the *gross* (visible) tumor out." Only the pathologist, after looking at the tissue under the microscope, can make a definitive diagnosis of cancer. And only the pathologist can tell you whether *all the cancer is out*. If the pathologist says no tumor cells are seen at the margin, he or she actually is saying that, allowing for the limits of the microscope, probably no cancer cells are left behind in the patient. If the pathologist notices cancer cells at the margin of the tissue, some cancer cells may have been left behind, implying that all the cancer has not been removed. The surgeon (who does not have microscopic vision!) may not have seen these microscopic cells at the margin.

You can see on Decision Tree 3 that there are two types of open biopsies—an excisional biopsy or lumpectomy, as it is often inelegantly called, and an incisional biopsy. Which one you have will depend on your long-term goals.

The Excisional Biopsy

You've had a needle biopsy and the results were positive. You have breast cancer. If at all possible, you want to preserve your breast. An excisional biopsy (lumpectomy) is the way to go. Or your lump and the diagnostic mammogram are very suspicious. If you have decided on breast preservation, you might go directly to a lumpectomy. In this situation, if the lump turns out to be cancer, the lumpectomy can be diagnostic as well as therapeutic—part of the treatment.

Let's say that the pathologist confirms breast cancer. In an excisional biopsy, only the suspicious area plus a rim of normal tissue is removed. Think of an egg in a frying pan. The yolk is the cancer surrounded by the white of the egg, which represents the rim of surrounding normal tissue. Optimally, the yolk is roughly centered and entirely surrounded by the eggwhite. If the yolk is off to one side or at the edge of the white and cut through, you have a problem.

Pathologists can see all this under the microscope. They call the outside edge of the rim of normal tissue (the white of the egg) the margin. If the pathologist calls the margin negative, or clear, that means there are no detectable cancer cells at the margin, that the excision has removed the entire cancer, and that it was surrounded by a rim of normal, noncancerous tissue. Ideal! You, the patient, are ready for the next step: the treatment team.

If, however, the pathologist sees cancer cells at the margin's edge, the margin is labeled positive. In this case, it is very likely that cancer cells remain behind in the breast, cells that could potentially grow and spread to other parts of the body. To avoid this dangerous situation, a reexcision may be necessary to ensure that no cancer cells remain at the edge of the tumor bed. Chapter 4 goes into more detail about how the pathologist describes the margins of a cancer.

Your surgeon carries out the reexcision in the operating room, since it is an open procedure. The biopsy site is clearly visible once the incision is made through the original scar. Additional tissue is scooped out of the biopsy site and again subjected to the pathologist's evaluation. If the reexcisional biopsy margins are negative, you can proceed to the next step in breast preservation.

However, if the biopsy margins continue to be positive after a re-excision, it is possible that the cancer does not have a distinct margin and that it spreads into the surrounding breast tissue. In this case, multiple excisional biopsies may never get negative margins without removing so much breast tissue that the breast is deformed. You should discuss with your treatment team the possibility of having a mastectomy, a procedure in which your entire breast is removed. This is an agonizing decision for most women, and your treatment team can be of immeasurable help. You may be willing to undergo a *third* procedure, a re-reexcision, to ensure negative margins. However, you should first talk over your prospects for breast preservation with your surgeon and the rest of your treatment team.

The Incisional Biopsy

Like an excisional biopsy, an incisional biopsy is an open procedure and is carried out in the operating room. Only a part of the lump is removed. An incisional biopsy is seldom carried out in preference to the needle biopsy, an office procedure.

You may or may not know from your core needle biopsy that your breast lump is cancer. In either case, you—and your doctors—may need more information about the type of cancer you may have. For example, if inflammatory breast is suspected, you need to know if the lymphatic ducts in the skin (dermal lymphatics) contain cancer cells. The needle biopsy may not answer such questions. An incisional biopsy may be necessary.

If the lump is cancer, you would expect the margins of an incisional biopsy to be positive. If, for example, the cancer is too large in proportion to the size of the breast for breast preservation to be feasible, a mastectomy is the treatment of choice. In that case, it doesn't matter if the margins of the biopsy are positive, because all the cancer probably will be excised when the breast is removed.

If the incisional biopsy is negative—that is, no cancer cells are found and the incisional biopsy is the first diagnostic procedure—it is possible that the specimen could be negative as a result of sampling error, and that cancer might be found in another part of the tumor. If your incisional biopsy is negative, your treatment team, including your pathologist, can help you determine whether the tumor is sufficiently suspicious to warrant reexcision of the entire tumor or a mastectomy.

If no cancer is found in your tumor, you should have another mammogram in one month and again in six months, and have your breast examined by your physician to be sure nothing is suspicious. If this is the case, you can resume the usual screening.

The Stereotactic Localization Excisional Biopsy

Suppose there is no palpable lump associated with the calcifications that are seen on the screening mammogram. *Some* of these calcifications may have been sampled stereotactically. If all of the calcifications are to be removed, the mammographer stereotactically localizes the calcifications as previously described. Once the calcifications have been localized, a wire or needle is placed in their midst. It extends from the calcifications in the breast to outside the breast, showing the surgeon where to place the incision. You, the patient, are then moved from the mammography suite to a surgical suite where the excision is carried out.

To surgically excise these calcifications, and because the calcifica-

tions are not associated with a lump that can be felt, the surgeon performs a needle localization biopsy (also known as a stereotactic biopsy).
By complex computerization the mammographer has localized the calcifications and placed a needle or a wire in the site to help the breast
surgeon find the specimen.

Since the excised tissue containing suspicious calcifications does
not feel significantly different from the surrounding tissue, the excised
specimen is generally mammogrammed to be sure that all the calcifications have been removed. This specimen mammogram is carried
out under the direction of the mammographer, generally back in the
mammography area. The mammographer, after examining the specimen, tells the surgeon whether all the calcifications were removed.

As you can see, it is necessary to schedule both the surgeon and
the mammographer for this complex procedure.

Remember . . .

- In general, when one has a biopsy, a piece of the tumor or all of the
  tumor is removed for examination under the microscope by the
  pathologist.
- The pathologist is the *only* specialist physician who is qualified to
  make the final, definitive diagnosis.
- There are two major categories of biopsy: the needle biopsy and the
  open biopsy.
- A needle biopsy has two primary advantages: (1) it is an outpatient
  procedure that can be carried out during an office visit to either a
  surgeon or a radiologist; (2) it can give a quick diagnosis of cancer
  when it is positive, thereby enabling you to explore the various approaches to treatment with greater certainty and eliminate a fruit-
  less period of anxiety.
- Anyone undergoing a needle biopsy should understand that it has

one serious disadvantage: a negative biopsy is not at all useful. It does not mean that cancer is *not* present. You are not out of the woods if you have a negative needle biopsy.

- There are two subcategories of needle biopsy: the fine-needle biopsy (FNA) and the core needle biopsy.

- There are two major categories of open biopsy: the excisional biopsy and the incisional biopsy.

- Both types of open biopsy are carried out in the operating room. They have the advantage of giving maximum information about your cancer. But they have the disadvantage that more time is involved in scheduling the procedure and ultimately in your surgeon's getting the pathologist's report and relaying the results to you. It is time that can make an already jittery patient even more jittery.

- If a woman diagnosed as having cancer of the breast decides to preserve her breast, the excisional biopsy—or lumpectomy—can be diagnostic as well as therapeutic.

- If an incisional biopsy is carried out, in which only a piece of the tumor is removed for study under the microscope, the margins probably will be positive. The incisional biopsy is performed as a diagnostic procedure and when there is little or no possibility of breast preservation.

Chapter 4   The Pathologist's Report

By this time you have received a diagnosis based on the biopsy findings. You know whether or not you have cancer. Your diagnosis was
made by the pathologist—the only member of your diagnostic team
whom you probably won't meet. In Chapter 3 you learned a good deal
about what a pathologist does, and about his or her role in a surgical
biopsy. Let's look now at what sort of report you can expect.

A cytopathologist issues a cytology report if you had a fine-needle
aspiration biopsy (FNA); a surgical pathologist issues a pathology report if you had any other kind of biopsy. A sample of each kind of
report appears at the end of this chapter. This chapter explains the information you should glean from your report. As with mammogram
and operation reports, you should be sure to get a copy of your cytology report and/or pathology report.

Cells, not tissue, are involved in an FNA. The cytology report should contain information on whether or not cells are present, and the character of the cells that are seen under the microscope.

A surgical pathology report may be in the form of a template or freely dictated, but either way it should contain certain information. Don't just read the summary of the findings at the end of the report. *Read and understand the body of the report.*

Look at the sample surgical pathology report at the end of this chapter. Note the separation of gross findings from microscopic findings. Although they are different, both are important to the final diagnosis. The "gross pathology" may be dictated by a different pathologist from the one who signs the report, because the gross pathology is done the day the specimen arrives in the pathology laboratory; the tissue is not read until it has been examined under the microscope by the pathologist who dictates the microscopic findings. The final surgical pathology report may not be typed and signed until days later.

The crucial information you should glean from the gross pathology is the size, location, and character of the specimen tissue as a whole, and the size, location, and character of the cancer (if there is any) that may be contained within it. Don't confuse the two. The larger dimensions of the specimen as a whole are *not* the dimensions of the cancer. The size of the cancer has major implications for the "stage" of the cancer.

If cancer is diagnosed within the specimen, the further description of the tissue, as set forth in the gross pathology, becomes important, including the location of the cancer within the specimen as a whole. For example, a pathologist often can make the diagnosis of inflammatory breast cancer when he or she sees, under the microscope, cancer cells in the lymphatic ducts of the skin—the "dermal lymphatics." As noted in Chapter 3, if the cancer is located on the edge of the specimen and is cut through, a reexcision will be necessary. The gross pathology has told the whole story. The microscopic pathology to come will simply confirm that the margin is positive (see Figure 6).

The color and the consistency of the tumor within the specimen are also relevant, in that they may characterize the tumor.

After dictating his or her findings, the pathologist who carries out the gross pathology will cut some of the tissue into small pieces and put them into "cassettes," porous holders of the fragments. The cassettes are submerged in a fluid that preserves the tissue. Please note that the pathologist cannot examine every cell in a core needle specimen, or in the larger specimen of an open biopsy. He or she may "bread loaf" the tissue by cutting it into slices like a loaf of bread and putting representative sections into cassettes. The remainder of the specimen is retained in jars containing preserving liquid, so that if there are any questions regarding the pathology, additional tissue can be examined. Legally, the pathology department must keep the preserved tissue for a specified period; nothing should be thrown away at the time of the procedure.

After an appropriate time, laboratory technicians prepare the preserved tissue further for the pathologist who will carry out the microscopic examination. They place very thin sections of the tissue on glass microscope slides, stain them appropriately, and cover them. The pathologist reads the slides under the microscope and dictates the "microscopic examination" portion of the report. The concluding summary gives the gist of the gross and microscopic findings.

The most common breast cancer is called adenocarcinoma. The term is really a composite: "adeno" describes the tissue of origin of the cancer; "carcinoma" is a fancy term for cancer. Thus, an adenocarcinoma is a cancer of glandular origin. And a breast adenocarcinoma is a breast cancer of glandular origin.

The specific tissue where the breast cancer has originated is either

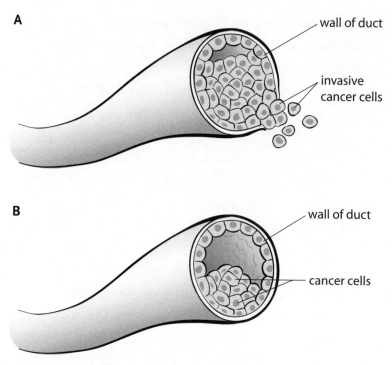

Figure 5 A, This diagram of invasive breast cancer shows that the cancer cells have spread outside the duct and invaded nearby breast tissue. *B,* This diagram of noninvasive breast cancer illustrates both ductal carcinoma in situ (DCIS) and lobular carcinoma in situ (LCIS). *Source:* National Cancer Institute.

in the duct system of the breast (when it is known as ductal adenocarcinoma or, more commonly, ductal carcinoma) or in the lobules (the part of the breast system where the milk is produced).

Lobular carcinomas, when invasive, have a life expectancy similar to that of invasive ductal carcinomas (Figure 5A). Although they may have different characteristics, the two are subjected to the same treatment. (You should be aware that invasive lobular carcinomas frequently are not visualized on screening mammograms because, it is believed, their outside edges have more tendrils and are not distinct.)

Both ductal and lobular carcinomas are treated differently when they are noninvasive (Figure 5B) than when they are invasive. A noninvasive ductal carcinoma (otherwise known as a DCIS, an acronym for ductal carcinoma in situ) has a different treatment path from that of a lobular carcinoma in situ, LCIS. Decision Tree 5, in Chapter 6, shows the treatment paths for the two forms of noninvasive breast cancer.

The report dictated by the pathologist is typed and submitted to him or her for approval and signature. Finally, it is conveyed to you. You can see why it takes several days to issue the pathology report, and several more days until you get the results. Your physician may wish to shorten the time involved by phoning the pathologist and getting an oral report. But if you then get the report from the physician, who did not see the tissue under the microscope, it is certainly possible for error to creep into the transmission.

When you receive the formal report, read all of it, not just the summary. If you don't understand the details, ask your doctor to explain them. Pathologists should know all about the tissue they are handling, including the "natural history" (untreated history) of the tumor. The report will contain the answers to three big questions: Do you have cancer? If so, what kind is it? And especially, is it invasive or noninvasive? The pathologist's answers will have profound consequences for your treatment.

If the margin is positive, the pathologist should be able to say how positive it is. As you can see from Figure 6, the margin can be "grossly" positive (many, many cancer cells are there) or "diffusely" positive (only a relatively few cells can be seen). Obviously, if the yolk is off center, at the edge of the white of the egg, and is cut through, the margin will be called grossly positive. In fact, if the tumor has been cut through, a large number of cancer cells will remain in the tumor bed (the remaining tissue in *you*). Although it is important for your team to know if the margin is grossly or diffusely positive, the bottom line for you is that if the margin is called positive, further surgery—a reexcision of the margin of the tumor bed—must be considered.

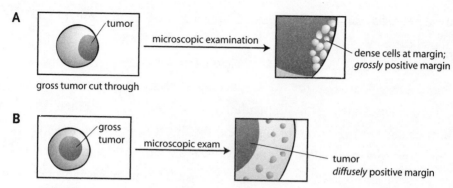

Figure 6 A, Diagram of a grossly positive margin, where the tumor has been cut through. The margin is also microscopically positive, as expected. B, Diagram of a diffusely positive margin, where the tumor is grossly distant from the margin. Nonetheless, microscopic examination shows some tumor cells at the margin.

If the pathologist's report after your biopsy describes cells in the lymphatics of the skin, you have a diagnosis of inflammatory breast cancer. If that specialized cancer is treated like plain old breast cancer (POBC), the outcome can be disastrous. Any suspicion of inflammatory breast cancer must be followed up, with a second opinion from another pathologist or oncologist if necessary. Unlike the treatment for POBC (surgery, chemotherapy or hormonal therapy, and radiation), the sequence of treatment for inflammatory breast cancer is chemotherapy or hormonal therapy first, then surgery, and then radiation. If inflammatory breast cancer is treated with a mastectomy at the outset, the cancer cells in the dermal lymphatics are cut through at the time of the initial surgery and can spread all over the chest wall. Soon thereafter, cancer nodules can appear on the chest wall *en curasse*—covering the entire chest wall. This progression spells disaster for the patient.

If chemotherapy or hormonal therapy can render the dermal lymphatics free of cancer, there are two results. First, the peau d'orange appearance of the breast skin can disappear and, second, surgery can be carried out safely. At the same time, the systemic therapy affects the large central mass of tumor and makes it much smaller, and therefore surgically amenable to treatment.

The pathologist has still another role: to give the cancer a pathologic stage. This final and crucial staging has a significant bearing on your future. The pathologist never makes formal treatment recommendations, because the pathologist is not a treating physician. The treatment team makes treatment *recommendations*. Only the patient makes treatment *decisions*.

The pathologist may have a strong opinion about what the treatment should be, but it is not stated in the pathology report or in any formal setting in which the pathologist participates (for example, at a tumor board—about which you will hear more in a moment). If the disease or tumor diagnosed is rare, the pathologist may comment appropriately in the pathology report.

Patients are usually pleased to have their case presented to a tumor board. They imagine that physicians with different specialties will carefully evaluate their case. The operative word is *carefully*.

Optimally, the slides should be presented by the pathologist assigned to the tumor board as well as by the presenting physician. Presumably the pathologist has had time to review the slides beforehand. Similarly, the x-rays should be evaluated prior to the tumor board meeting and presented by the assigned radiologist. If the slides and x-rays are carefully reviewed and presented, the role of the tumor board can be extremely meaningful.

Frequently, however, the films or slides are not present. Or the pathologist or radiologist is absent. Or the specialists have not had enough time to review the slides or films. Often the attending physician is seeing the slides for the first time. In such hit-or-miss circumstances, the board's recommendations may not be very thoughtful or they may be biased in favor of the presenting physician.

Even if the tumor board is well organized and well prepared, the case frequently is presented rather quickly. The pathologist, the radiologist, and the physicians on the board have little opportunity to think about the case, the patient is not seen, and the recommendations may be tainted by the presentation. There is no substitute for seeing and examining the patient and taking sufficient time to think about the case after reviewing all the records, films, and slides. Tumor board recommendations are just that—recommendations. They should never be accepted as definitive treatment decisions. Your treatment team is responsible for explaining your treatment options to you, and only you can decide what treatment you will have.

Remember . . .

- Only the pathologist, the member of your diagnostic team whom you probably will never see, makes the diagnosis of cancer.
- As with your x-ray reports and your operation report, you should ask for and receive your cytology and/or pathology report.
- A pathology report is divided into three parts: (1) the gross pathology, (2) the microscopic pathology, and (3) a summary of the findings. *Don't just read the summary.* You could miss crucial information.
- Many steps need to be taken in the pathology laboratory before the typed report becomes available. These steps take time—often many days.
- The breast cancers most commonly diagnosed are adenocarcinomas, ductal and lobular. Both forms can be invasive (infiltrating) or noninvasive.
- Even well-qualified physicians participating in a tumor board cannot make careful recommendations if they do not spend enough time to study all the films and slides. Even then, there is no substitute for examining the patient.

Sample Cytopathology Report

Patient: xxxxxxxxxxxxxxxxxxxxxxxxxxxxx

DOB/Age: xx/xx/xxxx (Age 45)

Gender: F

MRN: xxxxxxxx

Location: xxxxxxxx

Client: xxxxxxxx

Dept/Div: xxxxxxxx

Accession #: xxxxxxxx

Procedure Date: xx/xx/xx

Received: xx/xx/xx

Reported: xx/xx/xx

Physician(s): xxxxxxxx

Pathologist(s): xxxxxxxx

DIAGNOSIS:

Breast, right, fine-needle aspiration: Benign cyst.

Comment:

The aspirate consists of benign ductal cells, apocrine metaplasic, foam cells, and cellular debris.

Provided Clinical History:

Right-breast aspiration.

Gross Examination:

Received 2cc cloudy tan fluid. Prepared 1 fixed, 1 dry cytospin slide.

Sample Surgical Pathology Report

Patient: xxxxxxxxxxxxxxxxxxxxxxxxxxx[a]

DOB/Age: xx/xx/xxxx (Age 42)

Gender: F

MRN: xxxxxxx

Location: xxxxxxxx

Client: xxxxxxxx

Dept/Div: xxxxxxxx

Accession #: xxxxxxxx

Procedure Date: xx/xx/xx

Received: xx/xx/xx

Reported: xx/xx/xx

Physician(s): xxxxxxxx

  cc: Tumor Registry xxxxxxxx

Pathologist(s): xxxxxxxx

Comment:

1) The sentinel lymph node was large and was therefore submitted in two blocks. Keratin immunostains were performed on both blocks.

2) In the initial excision (part 2), carcinoma lies extremely close to the deep margin; however, since no additional tumor was identified in the reexcised deep margin tissue (part 3), all final margins are considered widely clear (greater than 0.5 cm). The patient's prior stereotactic needle core biopsy of this lesion (S03-18693) is noted.

Results to Dr. — via voicemail xx/xx/xx.

Provided Clinical History:

Left-breast cancer.

[a] This patient initially was diagnosed with breast cancer by a core needle biopsy. At the time of this surgery, the lump and the sentinel lymph node were removed. Because the margins of the excised tumor were regarded as "positive or close," a reexcision of the tumor bed was carried out.

Gross Examination:[b]

1) Received fresh labeled with the patient's ID and "left sentinel node" is a 2.8 x 1.7 x 0.6 cm fragment of adipose tissue containing a blue stained 1.8 x 0.4 x 0.5 cm crescentic lymph node. The node is bisected and then further divided, and entirely submitted on two chucks. The frozen section remnants are submitted as 1FSA and 1FSB.

2) Received fresh, labeled with the patient's ID and "left breast mass," is a 11.8 gm, 4.8 x 3.4 x 1.4 cm, oriented needle localization excision of fibrofatty breast tissue with surface blue dye staining. A specimen radiograph is included and has been interpreted as "Clip is specimen. DK." As per surgeon, wire is inferior and the blue staining is lateral. The specimen is inked as follows: superficial/lateral = blue, superficial/medial = green, deep/superior = black, and deep/inferior = yellow. The specimen is serially sectioned from lateral to medial revealing an ill-defined, 1.4 x 1.2 x 0.9 cm, firm, white fibrous area that abuts the deep margin. A 0.4 x 0.4 x 0.9 cm area of probable collagen plug is noted within the fibrous mass. The remaining surrounding breast tissue is primarily fatty. All of the fibrous tissue is sequentially submitted from medial to lateral in cassettes 2A-2F. The lateral-most fatty tissue is submitted in cassette 2I.

[b] The excised mass of tissue was maximally 4.8 cm. The tumor itself, on the other hand, measures 0.8 cm (taking into account the collagen plug that was seen). The size of the tumor is noted in the summary and also is represented in the TNM stage. *This is a classic example in which the specimen size is different from the tumor size.* The final diagnosis and stage of this patient can be found in the Template Summary at the end of the report.

3) Received in formalin, labeled with the patient's ID, and designated "reexcision deep margin," is a 4.6 gm, 4.1 x 2.3 x 0.8 cm, oriented fragment of fibroadipose breast tissue. A suture marks the anterior (old) margin as per surgeon. The old margin is inked yellow, and the new (deep) margin is inked black. The tissue is serially sectioned revealing a 0.2 x 0.5 cm area of possible collagen plug vs. fibrosis centrally. No other focal lesions are identified. The tissue is entirely submitted sequentially in cassettes 3A-3F.

Microscopic Examination:
Performed.

Intraoperative Examination:
1) Present Section Diagnosis, left sentinel node—no evidence of malignancy, one node.
2) Stat Gross Diagnosis, left breast tissue—Deep margin extremely close to tumor.

Diagnosis:
1) Sentinel lymph node, left axillary, excision:
       A) No evidence of malignancy, 1 node.
       B) Keratin immunostains negative.

2,3) Left breast, excisional biopsy with reexcision of deep margin:

Template Summary

TUMOR HISTOLOGIC TYPE: Infiltrating ductal carcinoma.
TUMOR LOCATION: Left breast.
TUMOR SIZE: 0.8 cm.
DCIS COMPONENT: Grade 2/3, 5% of lesion.

Sample Surgical Pathology Report, continued

TUMOR GRADE (modified BSR): 6/9

      Tubule Formation: 2/3

      Nuclear Grade: 2/3

      Mitotic Activity: 2/3

ANGIOLYMPHATIC INVASION: Absent.

MARGINS: Final margins widely clear.

MICROCALCIFICATIONS: Absent.

SKIN/NIPPLE INVOLVEMENT: Not submitted/Not submitted.

ER/PR: Positive/Positive (by immunostains).

HER-2/NEU: Negative for overexpression of HER-2/neu oncogene protein by immunostains.

LYMPH NODES: No evidence of malignancy, 1 sentinel node (part 1).

PATHOLOGIC STAGE (TNM): pT1b N0 MX.

Chapter 5 Your Treatment Team and Second Opinions

The radiologist/mammographer has read your mammograms, the surgeon and/or a mammographer has carried out your biopsy, and the pathologist has looked at your biopsy specimen under the microscope and given you the final diagnosis. These three specialists constitute your *diagnostic* team. Although you may have met the first two and will probably never meet the third, each specialist is critically important to your care (Box 7). A mistake by any one of them could have profound consequences for you. That is why it is essential to select well-trained, experienced physicians as well as an excellent hospital where, for example, high-quality pathology is carried out. Your very life could depend on the interpretation of your biopsy by the pathologist, *the specialist you never see.*

If you do not have cancer, your care very likely will end here. But if you are diagnosed to have cancer, another team of specialists, the *treatment* team, will take over your care.

Decision Tree 4 The Treatment Team

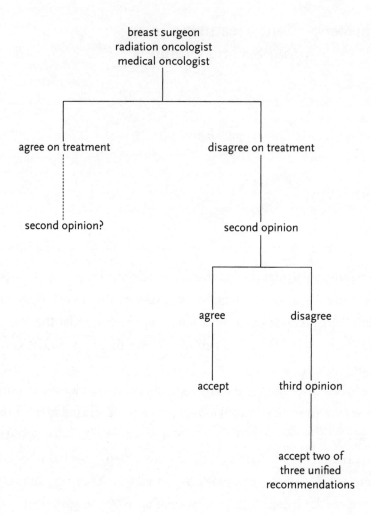

breast surgeon
radiation oncologist
medical oncologist

agree on treatment   disagree on treatment

second opinion?   second opinion

agree   disagree

accept   third opinion

accept two of
three unified
recommendations

Box 7 Training of Breast Cancer Specialists

This category includes breast radiologists, breast pathologists, breast surgeons, breast radiation oncologists, and breast
medical oncologists. Each has an M.D. degree and has spent
many years in post-doctoral training to pass the specialty board
examinations in his or her particular field.

The training of a breast cancer expert may go beyond the
board requirements of the specialty field. For example, a breast
surgeon spends six to seven years as an intern and a resident
after receiving the M.D. degree. He or she then passes general
surgical board exams, which credential this individual as a general surgeon. Next is the board examination in surgical oncology, which is the highest board exam that must be passed. He
or she may take a breast surgical fellowship. It is possible to
limit one's practice to breast surgery; however, few surgeons
can afford this kind of restriction. Most also carry out general
surgical procedures or general cancer surgical procedures.

Similarly, radiologists, pathologists, and radiation oncologists must pass specialty board exams after their internship
and residency. Medical oncologists generally take boards in
internal medicine after completing an internal medicine residency. They must then spend an additional two years in a
hematology/oncology fellowship and pass these exams as well.

Any of these physicians may become specialists in breast
cancer and restrict their clinical activities accordingly. Thus,
radiologists become mammographers, and those in the other
specialties become similarly specialized by limiting their clinical activity to breast cancer.

Do You Need a Second Opinion?

Be sure you are satisfied that you have the correct diagnosis before you make the transition to treatment. *When a diagnosis of cancer is involved, never fear that you will hurt the feelings of any of your doctors if you ask for a second opinion.* Competent physicians will never object, as long as the second opinion is obtained from a reputable physician (or group of physicians). In fact, competent physicians appreciate having their opinion verified by outside physician-experts. Pathologists, for example, are often asked by treating physicians to send their specimens to other pathologists for confirmation of the diagnosis. At any time during your care, if you have questions or doubts about your diagnosis or about treatment recommendations, you should ask for a second opinion. Your life is at stake and you need to be sure you are making appropriate decisions based on an accurate diagnosis.

Your Treatment Team

Once you are satisfied with the diagnosis, you should go over all the options of your treatment with *each* member of your treatment team. This team consists of a breast surgeon (possibly the same one who carried out your breast biopsy), a radiation oncologist (one who treats cancer with radiation), and a medical oncologist (one who treats cancer with chemotherapy, hormonal therapy, or biologics—systemic therapy). *Be sure that your treatment team has designed an approach specifically for your treatment.* Although you may feel you already know which course of treatment you prefer to undertake, your treatment team may have a different recommendation based on experience and information. Listen carefully to each of your doctor-specialists. If your case is not particularly complex, all three should agree, at least in principle, on the appropriate treatment for you.

Even if a particular modality (surgery, radiation, or systemic therapy) is not included in the recommended treatment, it is important to get the opinion of *each* of the three specialists who constitute your treatment team. Each brings a different perspective based on his or her specialty. If you, the patient, have *any* questions or concerns about their recommendations, you should seek another opinion from another reputable team. If the opinions of the two teams differ, seek a third opinion from still another reputable group. Two of the three opinions should agree, not necessarily in detail but definitely in principle, regarding which treatment or treatments are needed and the sequence that should be followed.

Let's say that you have been diagnosed with infiltrating ductal carcinoma, T2, NO, MO (stage II). "Infiltrating" is the pathologist's word for "invasive." Thus, you have a breast cancer measuring between two and five centimeters—say 2.3 centimeters. Your bra cup is size A or B. The surgeon says you need a mastectomy (removal of the breast) because the tumor is too large relative to the size of your breast; the radiation oncologist says you could have a lumpectomy followed by radiation (breast preservation); and the medical oncologist says you need chemotherapy to make the tumor smaller before you have any surgery (neoadjuvant chemotherapy). Your team does not agree; you need a second opinion from another competent, experienced team. Even if you have to travel out of town for it, and even if this second opinion is not covered by your health insurance, don't be deterred. *Get a competent second opinion from an experienced team.* And if this second opinion is not satisfactory, seek a third opinion. If your case is complex, even if your initial treatment team's recommendation is unanimous, you may still wish to get a second opinion to have that recommendation confirmed by another team.

Most cases are straightforward and members of the initial treatment team generally will agree and come up with a unified recommendation. If their conclusion seems reasonable to you, you may decide not to seek further opinions. The important thing is to be well enough informed that you are confident in your own decision making.

Remember . . .

- A *diagnostic team* is different from a *treatment team*.
- Even if you think you know which treatment approach you wish to take, be sure you have discussed your treatment with each member of your treatment team. One or more may have a different point of view, depending on the specialty represented. You need to hear *all* viewpoints before making your final decision.
- Competent physicians never object to second opinions.
- Your diagnosis should never be in doubt. If it is, seek a second, or even a third, opinion.
- Your treatment should never be in doubt. If it is, seek a second, or even a third, opinion.
- If you seek a second opinion, the two treatment teams should agree on their recommendations after they have reviewed all the data accumulated on your case. If the two teams disagree, you may have to seek a third opinion. You should obtain agreement by two teams, especially if your case is complex. If your case is straightforward, you may wish to accept the reasonable recommendation of your initial treatment team and not require another opinion.
- Second and third opinions should be obtained from competent, experienced physicians or groups of physicians—experts in their fields.
- If your insurance does not cover a second or third opinion, please spend the money to get a second opinion from a competent group of breast cancer experts. Your life and your quality of life are crucial. You are worth the expense.

Chapter 6　Surgery and Staging of Your Breast Cancer

If you were diagnosed with breast cancer between 1900 and the late 1970s, you were referred to a surgeon and you had the only available procedure, which in those days was a radical mastectomy. You did not need a decision tree. You did not need a treatment team. If you grew up during that time, or if you read the statistics on breast cancer during those years, you know that women who were newly diagnosed to have breast cancer were diagnosed in the late stages of the disease and often had little chance of recovery. They had either locally advanced breast cancer or metastatic breast cancer.

Today breast cancer is being diagnosed at an early stage and is potentially curable (Figure 7). Research has given us numerous options for treatment, and more are on the way. Now there *is* need for a decision tree and for a treatment team.

As Decision Tree 5 shows, your surgeon has three functions: (1) to diagnose breast cancer, (2) to treat breast cancer, and (3) to surgically stage the axillary (underarm) lymph nodes. *Your* first treatment deci-

Decision Tree 5 Surgical Options

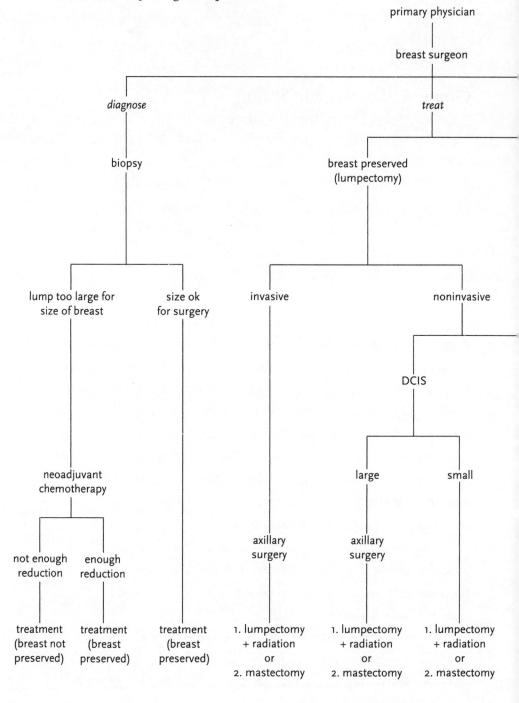

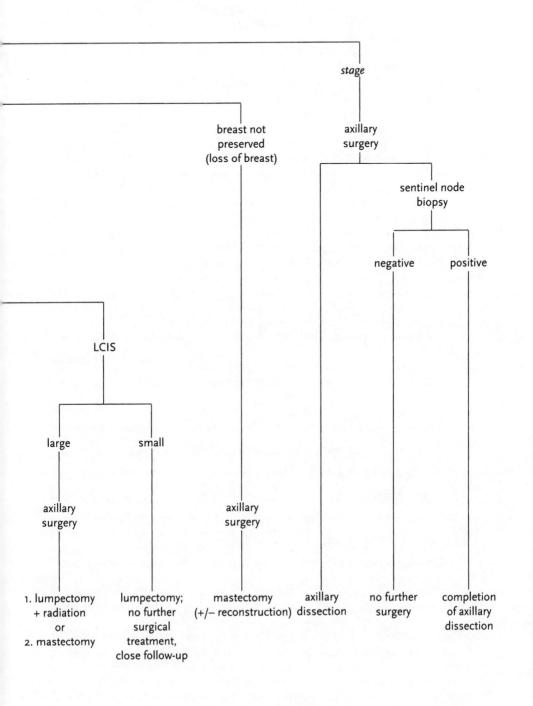

stage

breast not
preserved
(loss of breast)

axillary
surgery

sentinel node
biopsy

negative   positive

LCIS

large   small

axillary
surgery

axillary
surgery

1. lumpectomy
+ radiation
or
2. mastectomy

lumpectomy;
no further
surgical
treatment,
close follow-up

mastectomy
(+/− reconstruction)

axillary
dissection

no further
surgery

completion
of axillary
dissection

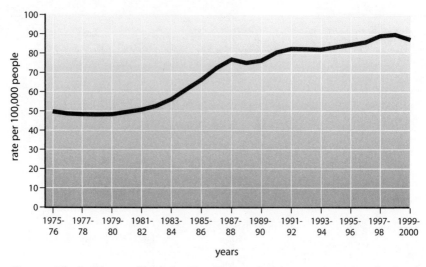

Figure 7 The incidence of early localized breast cancer over time. Very few local-ized breast cancers were seen between 1975 and 1987; most cases of breast can-cer seen in those years were advanced. The trend was reversed by the year 2000, when most breast cancers diagnosed were localized.

sion is between preserving your breast and losing it—undergoing a mastectomy. This basic choice probably will not change substantially for many years. In either case, your treatment will start with surgery.

The surgeon may or may not be the same person who performed your biopsy, but a surgeon should be part of the treatment team you have chosen. A treatment plan, including decisions related to systemic therapy and radiation, should be in place *before* you have further treat-ment for breast cancer. If an unexpected adverse event occurs, and it often does, you will have discussed the possibilities with your doctors and will have a plan for how to deal with them.

Of course, your treatment may have already begun if you had an excisional biopsy, because that is what a lumpectomy is. Ideally, if you had an excisional biopsy, before the operation you chose the other members of your treatment team (in close coordination with your di-agnostic team) and discussed your provisional treatment plan with all of them. It should be clear to everyone involved that your goal is to preserve your breast.

In addition to performing the treatment lumpectomy or mastectomy, your surgeon will surgically stage your axilla. This will be a separate operation if your biopsy derived from your lumpectomy; if not, the two procedures can be performed at the same time. Then, after your pathologist has confirmed the stage of your cancer (pathologic staging), you will be ready for the postsurgical phases of your treatment.

Primary Surgery for Breast Cancer

Breast Preservation

Your breast surgeon is your first *treating* physician and, along with the other members of your treatment team, will help you make the choice between breast preservation (often called breast conservation) and a mastectomy as the primary treatment for your breast cancer.

If you have chosen breast preservation, lumpectomy followed by radiation will constitute your primary treatment. The size of your tumor will determine whether a lumpectomy can be carried out immediately. If, for example, the tumor is too large for the size of your breast (a five-centimeter mass in a size A breast), an attempt may be made to reduce the size of the tumor with neoadjuvant chemotherapy. Most tumors shrink with chemotherapy. If there is not enough shrinkage, you still will need a mastectomy. If the tumor shrinks adequately, a lumpectomy can be carried out, thereby preserving the breast. Sometimes the tumor even disappears altogether.

"Excisional biopsy," "wide excision," "lumpectomy," "partial mastectomy"—these terms are all different names for the same procedure. Each means removal of the cancerous tissue in your breast as well as a surrounding rim of normal tissue. The term "lumpectomy" is inelegant, but it seems to have been accepted by the lay community

and now is the term most used, even among doctors. "Partial mastectomy" is the term favored by many surgeons and pathologists, to distinguish the procedure from a modified radical mastectomy (removal
of the breast and the first two levels of draining lymph nodes) or a
simple mastectomy (removal of the breast without removal of any
lymph nodes). It is *not* a "quadrantectomy," in which a quadrant (one
fourth) of the breast is removed. That operation is very deforming, especially after several years, and is not commonly used in the United
States. Be sure you and your breast surgeon understand exactly the
procedure you want to have, as well as the side on which the procedure is to be carried out.

An experienced breast surgeon knows where and how to localize
the scar for your lumpectomy so that it will not deform your breast
and will be unobtrusive. Furthermore, he or she also knows how to
use a plastic surgical technique for closing the tissues so that suture
marks are not visible (Figure 8).

If no previous biopsy has determined whether your cancer is invasive or noninvasive, you will learn that now, when the pathologist reports the findings on the lumpectomy specimen. As you can see on
Decision Tree 5, this determination will affect whether axillary lymph
node surgery will need to be performed, as well as whether you will
need radiation. Indirectly, it also determines whether you will need
systemic therapy. But your basic choice will still be whether or not to
preserve your breast.

Both the breast surgeon and the radiation oncologist who will
give you your postoperative radiation treatments require special training and equipment to successfully carry out the technique of breast
preservation. If they do not have access to both, try to find a facility
where they do. If you cannot travel to where the appropriate expertise
is available, do not have the procedure. It is preferable to have a mastectomy than to have poor breast preservation.

A   B

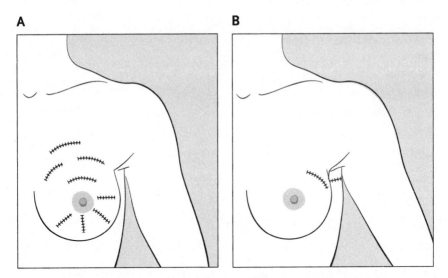

Figure 8 A, This recommended placement of incisions for breast preservation surgery will result in curved scars in the upper half of the breast, and linear scars in the lower half. Both short-term and long-term deformities of the breast are thereby minimized. *B,* The breast lumpectomy is usually carried out first. The axillary nodes are removed as a separate procedure, with a different incision. *Source:* Adapted from NSABP's "Recommended Incisions for Breast Conservation Treatment."

Mastectomy

Mastectomy is the loss of the entire breast, including the nipple and its surrounding areola (the pinkish to brownish tissue that surrounds the nipple). Although today most women try to preserve their breast, many still have a mastectomy. From a medical standpoint, a mastectomy may be the only sound choice. Or a mastectomy may be selected for a variety of other reasons. Perhaps the patient is fearful of radiation; or she may not wish to have the prolonged treatment that breast preservation requires. You should know, however, that in the hands of a competent breast surgeon, a mastectomy need not be disfiguring.

As with lumpectomy, a competent breast surgeon leaves a single horizontal, thin scar, which has been closed with appropriate plastic

Figure 9 Scar from a modified radical mastectomy. Note that it extends laterally because the axillary lymph nodes have been removed through the same incision.

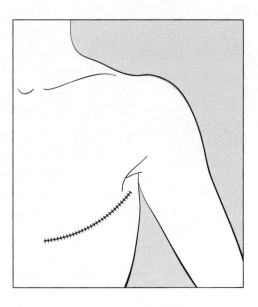

surgical technique and therefore does not show any suture marks (Figure 9). The tissue should be pulled tightly enough that there is not a lot of redundant tissue, unless later reconstruction is planned.

It is best to make a decision about breast reconstruction before the mastectomy. The breast surgeon and the plastic surgeon can then consult with each other beforehand so that the appropriate technique is carried out at the time of the mastectomy. You yourself should be sure that they do consult and that you know how the procedure will be carried out.

The several different types of mastectomy range from the most to the least drastic. Today, a radical mastectomy is rarely performed. It was the procedure of choice until the late 1970s, when a National Cancer Institute consensus report indicated that survival and recurrence rates were essentially the same for modified radical mastectomy and for radical mastectomy, stage for stage. The modified radical mastectomy, a far less disfiguring and invasive surgery, became the prevailing treatment and remains so at the present time.

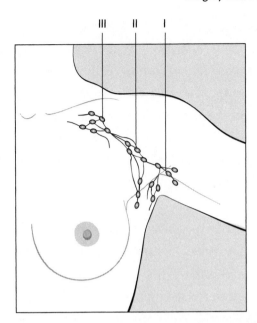

III   II   I

Figure 10 Level I, II, and III axillary lymph nodes. One major difference between a modified radical mastectomy and a radical mastectomy is the removal of level I and II lymph nodes in the modified radical mastectomy as opposed to the removal of all three levels in a radical mastectomy.

A modified radical mastectomy includes removal of the lower two levels of lymph nodes in your axilla instead of the three levels removed in a radical mastectomy, plus the involved breast (Figure 10). The breast surgeon follows strict surgical guidelines in carrying out the procedure. Removal of the breast, its nipple-areolar complex, and the first two levels of lymph nodes that drain the breast (levels I and II, found in the axilla of the arm) is routine. As much breast tissue as possible is removed from under the remaining skin of the chest wall without compromising the healing of the skin. (A small amount of breast tissue is necessarily left behind.) Again, in closing the wound, the surgeon uses a plastic surgical technique that does not show the sutures. The result is a single thin scar that crosses the chest wall horizontally and extends laterally so that the surgeon can carry out a standard lymph node dissection using the same incision (see Figure 9).

A "simple" mastectomy is one in which only the breast is removed, not the lymph nodes. The procedure is certainly not simple for the patient, but it is relatively simple for the surgeon—hence the name.

One other mastectomy procedure currently in vogue in some areas of the United States is the skin-sparing mastectomy. As the name suggests, the breast skin is conserved; not all of the skin of the breast is taken. Some surgeons say that in the skin-sparing mastectomy, if the margins are clear and the tumor is small and centrally placed, the skin is rarely the site of a recurrence. Nonetheless, a skin-sparing procedure should be recommended cautiously, and only after all the facts are known.

A competent breast surgeon uses *good judgment* and will not carry out any procedures that are not accepted as cancer surgery. Assume that a woman has opted for a mastectomy. She plans to have reconstructive surgery and wishes to preserve the nipple-areolar (NA) complex. The surgeon, wanting to please her, may attempt to preserve the nipple-areolar complex by moving it to a different location and then transferring it at a later time to the breast mound created by the plastic surgeon. *This is not a cancer operation.* Malignant breast cells might remain in the site in which the NA complex was initially located. To make matters worse, the NA complex itself might be contaminated with breast cancer cells, which may seed the reconstructed chest wall after the NA complex is again moved. The message is that you shouldn't try to talk your surgeon into nonstandard approaches to the surgical treatment of breast cancer.

Reconstruction

Although reconstruction is not a primary surgical treatment for breast cancer, it is an extremely important aspect of a mastectomy. Many women who have undergone a mastectomy, regardless of how long ago, state that they "feel whole again" after their chest wall has been reconstructed. For many women, planning a mastectomy is a much less distressing experience when they are simultaneously planning the reconstruction of their breast.

Reconstruction does not imply vanity. There is no reason to feel guilty because you wish to look as you did before your mastectomy. It is a normal, healthy feeling, and you should consider reconstruction if you're going to have a mastectomy.

Reconstruction can be carried out with any type of mastectomy. It can be done at the time of the mastectomy—this is known as immediate reconstruction—or any time afterward, even years after the mastectomy was performed.

Implants are used to create a breast mound. These implants have not been shown to cause cancer or to have serious untoward side effects. The plastic surgeon can discuss with you the type of implant recommended for your individual case. Also, he or she can explain how a nipple-areolar complex can be created later.

Other forms of reconstruction do not have some of the disadvantages of plastic implants. One is known as a TRAM-flap type of breast reconstruction because it involves the creation of a breast mound from the patient's own abdominal tissue. It is a much more complicated surgery than the usual implant type of reconstruction. Ask the plastic surgeon who recommends a TRAM-flap procedure how many successful cases he or she has done. Since not everyone is a candidate for a TRAM flap, find out from your physicians if the procedure is appropriate for you.

Another frequently used type of reconstruction using your own tissue is known as the lastissimus dorsi flap, which has evolved over the years and become popular in certain parts of this country. It is still major surgery although a significantly lesser procedure than the TRAM flap.

Always feel free to ask your surgeon, whether a breast surgeon or a plastic surgeon, if you can meet any of the patients who have had these various procedures. Talking with and seeing these women can help you with your own decision.

In general, health insurance companies will cover most, if not all, of the cost of reconstruction if it can be shown that the mastectomy was performed to treat breast cancer. After all, reconstruction is essentially the completion of the mastectomy.

Surgical Treatment of Invasive and Noninvasive Breast Cancer

You have learned from your pathology report whether your breast cancer is invasive or noninvasive. Only the pathologist can make that diagnosis after examining your breast specimen under the microscope.

If the cancer is invasive, axillary lymph node surgery must be carried out. However, if the cancer is noninvasive, whether or not you will need axillary surgery depends on the type of noninvasive cancer you have (Box 8 and see Decision Tree 5).

On Decision Tree 5, you can see that both forms of invasive breast cancer are treated similarly. Regardless whether it is invasive ductal or invasive lobular cancer, and whether you choose breast preservation or mastectomy, the lymph nodes under your arm (axillary lymph nodes) must be surgically explored to determine whether the cancer has spread there.

The two forms of noninvasive cancer are treated differently. If you have noninvasive ductal carcinoma, or DCIS, whether you choose breast preservation or mastectomy, you won't need axillary surgery unless the cancer is large. Exploration of the axilla generally is not regarded as necessary because if the noninvasive ductal carcinoma is small and the pathologist confirms that there is no detectable invasion, the likelihood that the cancer has spread to the axillary lymph nodes is vanishingly slim. For the same reason, systemic therapy will not be offered to anyone with a small DCIS. As you can see on Decision Tree 5, the noninvasive DCIS must be removed either by a lumpectomy or a

Box 8 Evolution of Treatment for Ductal Carcinoma
In Situ and Lobular Carcinoma In Situ

In the past, both DCIS and LCIS were treated with a mastectomy. In addition, women with LCIS were subjected to a "mirror image biopsy" (removal of tissue from the mirror image of their other, contralateral breast) even when there was no evidence of abnormality in the second breast! Because LCIS was very rarely found in the mirror image, this practice finally was stopped.

In the early 1980s, resistance to breast preservation for noninvasive breast cancer persisted. At one memorable meeting, a well-known breast surgeon stated that it seemed ridiculous to him that we were still performing mastectomies on women with *noninvasive* breast cancers while we were carrying out breast preservation on women with *invasive* breast cancer. This comment represented a turning point. Soon afterward, women with DCIS were given the choice between breast preservation with lumpectomy plus radiation, or mastectomy. Subsequent clinical trials showed the two treatments to be equivalent. Eventually lumpectomy followed by radiation became the norm.

The tide changed for LCIS as well. It was determined that LCIS took a very long time—on the order of eighteen years—to become invasive if left untreated. As a result, nowadays only a very wide surgical excisional biopsy is recommended for women with LCIS. Typically, all that they need after their lumpectomy is frequent, careful physical examinations and very frequent mammograms.

mastectomy. As in invasive breast cancer, a lumpectomy must be followed by radiation to complete the primary treatment.

The decision tree shows that if you have a small lobular carcinoma in situ, or LCIS, you won't even need radiation. For LCIS generally requires only a wide excisional biopsy with negative margins, followed by careful clinical breast exams and mammograms.

It's a different story if the noninvasive DCIS or LCIS is large, on the order of three to five or more centimeters. Even the most knowledgeable pathologist might miss some invasion in an apparently non-invasive cancer that large. In such cases I always recommend surgical exploration of the axilla. If any axillary nodes show cancer cells, one suspects some invasion was in the specimen. If the lymph nodes were positive, chemotherapy or hormonal therapy is recommended.

Axillary Lymph Node Surgery

If you are found to have invasive breast cancer, or if you fulfill any of the conditions that require surgical evaluation of your axillary lymph nodes, the axillary surgery takes place at the same time as your lumpectomy or mastectomy. There are two alternative methods of treating your axilla: a conventional axillary dissection (AD) or a sentinel node biopsy (SNB).

In either instance, surgical evaluation of your underarm (axillary) nodes must take place *before* further treatment. This procedure is part of the staging of your cancer. The status of your axillary lymph nodes not only will have predictive value, but will help determine the need for systemic therapy and even may influence the type of systemic therapy you have. Surgical evaluation of your axillary nodes completes the role of the surgeon in both treating and surgically staging your invasive breast cancer.

If you have a mastectomy with a conventional AD, the removal of the axillary contents does not necessarily require a separate incision. The lymph nodes can be removed at the same time as the breast, through the same horizontal incision—which crosses the chest wall after the breast has been removed.

What can you expect from the axillary surgery? If you decide on breast preservation, the axillary contents or the sentinel axillary lymph node(s) will be removed through a separate incision under your arm. This scar, like the breast scar, should be small and unobtrusive—generally placed in the natural fold of your axilla where it will be almost invisible.

Whether you have breast preservation or a mastectomy, the pathologist will examine the clump of tissue from under your arm to determine the stage of your cancer.

The Conventional Axillary Dissection

In a conventional axillary dissection (AD), level I and level II lymph nodes are removed in a pad of tissue excised from under your arm. Removal of these lower two levels of lymph nodes follows strict surgical guidelines and constitutes a "sampling" of the axillary lymph nodes. It is not a full axillary lymph node dissection—as in a radical mastectomy, where all three levels of axillary lymph nodes are removed (see Figure 10).

My patients often say, "I want to know exactly how many lymph nodes will be removed." Or I hear, "I want my surgeon to remove precisely x lymph nodes." The fact is, the breast surgeon cannot tell you in advance how many lymph nodes will be removed in the axillary dissection because of the guidelines on the removal of the lower two levels of lymph nodes contained in the pad of tissue under your arm. The tissue contains a variable number of lymph nodes, generally ranging between ten and twenty. Removal of fewer than ten lymph nodes during a standard AD is regarded by most breast cancer experts as an inadequate sampling of the nodes, a shortcoming that makes subsequent treatment decisions very difficult.

If the surgeon has adhered to the guidelines for a formal axillary dissection, the final count of the number of lymph nodes is in the hands of the pathologist. I recall a high of fifty-one lymph nodes that were counted in a pad of tissue containing the lower two levels. The high count resulted from the type of fluid used to prepare the tissue, as well as the diligence of the pathologist in counting the nodes. The tissue had been preserved in a special fluid that made even tiny lymph nodes visible. The high count did not mean that the patient had an excessive number of nodes in her axilla.

The Sentinel Node Biopsy

Surgeons have long been searching for ways to spare patients by subjecting them to less and less surgery, usually with fewer and fewer side effects. We have seen the transition from radical mastectomy to modified radical mastectomy to lumpectomy. The same sort of transition has taken place with the removal of axillary lymph nodes.

Surgeons have devised the sentinel node biopsy (SNB), a technique that removes only one to three lymph nodes from under the arm. This procedure has become the standard of care in many institutions for early-stage breast cancers, in spite of concern that adoption of SNB without adequate clinical trials to point the way may have been premature. Only time will tell.

The SNB is based on the following logic: A sentinel node is the first lymph node to drain the cancer in your breast, hence the term "sentinel." This sentinel node is purported to give as much information to an experienced pathologist as an examination of all the axillary nodes following conventional removal of the first two levels of lymph nodes. The assumption is that metastatic cancer cells have an orderly progression through the axillary lymph nodes. That is, they go first to the sentinel nodes, then beyond. If the sentinel node is negative, it is therefore presumed that the nodes downstream also will be negative. By the same token, if the sentinel node is positive, some of the downstream nodes will be positive over time. This procedure, the sentinel node biopsy, requires a separate scar in the axilla. But the scar can be smaller and even less obtrusive than the scar for conventional removal of level I and level II lymph nodes.

Overall, when one compares the SNB with the conventional AD, fewer adverse long-term side effects are associated with the former. This is to be expected, in that progressively lesser surgery—going from a radical mastectomy where all three levels of axillary lymph nodes are removed, to a modified radical mastectomy in which only the lowest two levels are removed—results in faster and better mobilization of the arm, as well as lower incidence of arm swelling. The removal of only the sentinel node(s) further reduces these complications.

The sentinel node biopsy potentially has two major advantages: (1) you can use your arm more quickly than if you have a conventional removal of level I and II nodes, and (2) your arm may not swell. However, we need more time to evaluate the long-term side effects of SNBs.

A sentinel node biopsy is carried out as follows. An inert blue dye and a radioactive solution (containing very little radioactive material) are injected into the tumor bed or lumpectomy site. After a specified period, the blue dye ends up in one node, the sentinel node. If the drainage is fast, however, the blue dye can end up in more than one node.

Since the radioactive solution travels the same pathway as the blue dye and the two accumulate together in the draining node(s), the radioactive solution is used to localize the blue node(s) in the axilla. The radiation can be detected by the surgeon *outside the skin* of the axilla by use of a small probe that is actually a Geiger counter. The surgeon then makes a small incision above the radioactive site, finds and removes the blue node(s), and submits the node(s) to the pathologist.

The surgeon's task is over. It is now the pathologist's turn. He or she carries out a meticulous examination of the blue node(s). If careful examination of the sentinel node reveals that any of the blue node(s) contain cancer, the surgeon later must surgically remove the remaining nodes as in a standard axillary node procedure. Actually a meticulous examination of the nodes can be accomplished at the time of surgery by means of a frozen section, which is a way of getting pathologic information rapidly, although not always accurately.

In rare instances, there is no uptake of blue dye in an axillary lymph node; the surgeon is then obliged to carry out a standard removal of the axillary nodes.

Clearly, you need both an experienced surgeon and an experienced pathologist to carry out a sentinel node biopsy successfully. If your surgeon is experienced but your pathologist is not, the sentinel biopsy that they carry out together is useless. Conversely, if your pathologist is experienced but your surgeon is not, the biopsy may be useless too.

Be sure to ask both the surgeon and the pathologist about their experience—how many SNBs and simultaneous conventional ADs they have performed. Each should have successfully completed twenty to thirty cases in which the SNB was carried out *simultaneously* with a standard AD. If in these twenty to thirty simultaneous procedures no pathologic difference was found in the number of involved nodes, these professionals are qualified to carry out the sentinel biopsy alone.

If you ask, your physician or your local American Cancer Society chapter can arrange for you to see patients who have undergone each of the surgical procedures described above. Through personal contact you can see the scars that you are considering. In fact, viewing these patients may help you make up your mind about which procedure you wish to have.

Staging Your Breast Cancer

The stage of your cancer must be accurately determined before treatment can continue. What does "stage" mean and what is its significance? The stage of a cancer indicates how far it has progressed: the size of the cancer in your breast, the presence or absence of cancer cells in your axillary lymph nodes, and whether or not your breast cancer has spread to other parts of your body. These three factors determine the *stage* of your breast cancer.

The surgeon's exploration of the axillary nodes, either by a conventional axillary dissection or by a sentinel node biopsy, concludes with surgical staging. The specimen goes to the pathologist, whose report tells whether there are any cancer cells in the lymph nodes and how many nodes contain cancer. Now a final pathologic stage can be assigned to your cancer.

The pathologic stage of your breast cancer will determine your prognosis, on a statistical basis. As I emphasize elsewhere in this book, *you* are not a statistic. I frequently hear patients say, "The doctors gave me three months to live, and here I am, six years later, alive and well." There is no refuting the fact that the lower the stage of breast cancer, the more likely it is that you can be cured. However, patients with higher stages, if they are not cured, can be *controlled* for long periods and, in these intervals, have a reasonable quality of life. Significant progress is being made in the treatment of breast cancer, and *you*, regardless of stage, may be the person who responds positively to a new advance. Time is an important factor. The longer you live, the greater the possibility that successful advances can be made to which you may respond positively.

What are the stages of breast cancer? Well, if the pathologist states that the size of your breast cancer is two centimeters or less, *and* you do not have positive axillary lymph nodes, *and* there is no indication that your cancer has spread elsewhere in your body, you have stage I breast cancer, which is potentially curable (Box 9).

If your breast cancer measures between two and five centimeters by pathology, you have stage II breast cancer, based on size alone. If, however, you are found to have a cancer that is less than two centimeters (a stage I size) *and* positive axillary lymph nodes—even one—you have stage II breast cancer based on the positive axillary node(s). In stage II breast cancer, the cancer has not spread beyond the breast and lymph nodes.

Stage III breast cancer consists of cancers that are equal to or greater than five centimeters in diameter and/or have positive axillary nodes that are clumped together—matted, we say. Although this is a large cancer, it is still localized because the cancer has not been shown to spread to other parts of the body.

Stage IV breast cancer, in contrast to stages I–III, is *not* localized. It is not confined to the breast and the draining lymph nodes. It has gone beyond the breast and axillary lymph nodes. Regardless of the size of the cancer or the axillary lymph node status, the stage is IV because the cancer can be found in distant sites. There has been metastasis.

Women with stage I to stage IV have *invasive* breast cancers.

Then there is stage 0. Patients who are stage 0 have *noninvasive* breast cancer. Their prognosis is excellent. No invasion can be found even after careful preparation of the tissue and a scrupulous examination under the microscope by the pathologist.

Metastatic Workup

I doubt you missed the term "metastasis" in the description of stage IV breast cancer. It's a word that people pay attention to. A metastasis refers to a cluster of cancer cells found at a distance from the original cancer. Under the microscope the metastasis looks distinctly like the original cancer and is found to be derived from the

Box 9 Staging Breast Cancer: The TNM system

T   *Primary Tumors*
To   Noninvasive ductal or lobular cancer (DCIS or LCIS)
T1   Tumor 2 centimeters or less in its greatest dimension
T2   Tumor more than 2 centimeters but not more than 5 centimeters in its greatest dimension
T3   Tumor equal to or more than 5 centimeters in its greatest dimension
T4   Tumor of any size with direct extension to chest wall or skin; includes inflammatory breast cancer

N   *Lymph Nodes under Arm*
No   No palpable lymph nodes under arm; regardless of whether axillary dissection or sentinel node biopsy, all lymph nodes studied under microscope are negative
N1   Lymph nodes studied under microscope contain tumor
N2   Axillary lymph nodes fixed to each other
N3   Lymph nodes around collar bone have tumor

M   *Distant Metastases*
Mo   No evidence of distant metastases
M1   Distant metastases present

Stage Grouping

Stage 0	To	No	Mo
Stage I	T1	No	Mo
Stage II	To	N1	Mo
	T1	N1	Mo
	T2	No, N1	Mo
Stage III	T1	N2	Mo
	T2	N2	Mo
	T3	No, N1, N2	Mo
Stage IV	T4	any N	any M
	any T	N3	any M
	any T	any N	M1

original cancer. If you hear that so-and-so has "bone cancer" or "brain cancer," it may be that the person has metastatic cancer to either bone or brain. If so, the cancer cells under the microscope are probably characteristic of the original tumor—not of bone or brain. (A cancer found to be characteristic of bone or brain is a *primary* tumor of the bone or brain.) If you have breast cancer and a metastasis is found in bone, it likely is not bone cancer, but breast cancer metastatic to bone. (By the same token, if a metastasis is found in the brain, it is not brain cancer, but rather metastatic breast cancer.)

The presence of a new metastasis often means that others may be lurking silently. Generally, the body is surveyed for other sites containing metastatic breast cancer. Such a survey is known as a metastatic workup. It comprises blood studies, x-rays (including a chest x-ray), bone scans (more sensitive than x-rays) to search for bone metastases, and, where appropriate, CT scans, MRIs, or PET scans. Positive bone scans are rarely found in women with stage I breast cancer. So, if you are found to have stage I breast cancer, do not expect to have a bone scan as part of a staging workup unless you have other symptoms suggesting that a scan is appropriate.

A metastatic workup should be carried out initially as part of staging. The presence of a metastasis, *discovered before treatment*, can change the treatment options.

Anyone who has undergone a metastatic workup knows the anxiety it produces. Breast cancer patients quickly learn that many metastases are silent and therefore their detection may be unexpected. The demonstration of metastatic disease can produce a cold sweat in the coolest of patients.

Sometimes metastatic disease is presumed to be present, even when its presence has not been proven. This is the case when axillary nodes are found to be positive. The presence of metastatic cells in the draining lymph nodes suggests, but doesn't prove, that cancer cells have left the primary site and have gone beyond the lymph nodes and escaped into the rest of the body, where they could grow into metastases.

Remember . . .

- Excisional biopsy, wide excision, lumpectomy, and partial mastectomy are essentially different names for the same procedure.
- An experienced breast surgeon knows where to place incisions and uses techniques to make the scars unobtrusive so they won't deform the breast.
- There are several types of mastectomy: a radical mastectomy, a modified radical mastectomy, a simple mastectomy, a skin-sparing mastectomy.
- Reconstruction should be considered if a mastectomy is recommended.
- It is important to know whether your tumor is invasive or noninvasive. The two require different treatments, as you can see in Decision Tree 5.
- The conventional axillary dissection and the sentinel node biopsy, fully described in this chapter, are different procedures with the same outcome.
- The staging of your breast cancer is critically important and will determine your treatment.
- Stage IV breast cancer is metastatic breast cancer. In this case, a metastatic workup is carried out. Treatment is based on symptoms.

Chapter 7 Radiation Therapy

Many patients are confused about the necessity for radiation after breast surgery. In your discussions with your treatment team before surgery, you may be so preoccupied with the surgery that all your questions are for your surgeon, and your surgeon may have tunnel vision about his or her own role. It may not occur to you to ask in detail about the treatment that follows. You may think that chemotherapy and radiation are equivalent *alternative* options. It's not uncommon to wonder, "If I have a lumpectomy and I have chemotherapy, do I then need radiation?" Or, "If I have a lumpectomy and radiation, do I then need chemotherapy?" In other words, can one therapy substitute for the other? Can chemotherapy replace radiation in my treatment for breast cancer? Or can radiation replace chemotherapy in the treatment for my breast cancer, since I don't want chemotherapy?

Before the surgical exploration of your axilla, neither you nor your doctors can be sure of the stage of your cancer. You may feel that you are in an emotional limbo. But once the stage is known, your post-

Decision Tree 6 Radiation

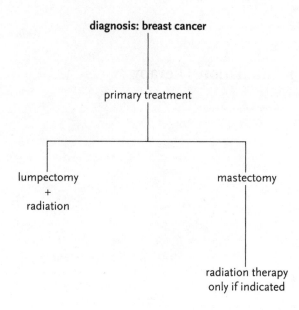

surgery treatment plan can be confirmed or modified, and set in motion.

Decision Tree 5 has shown you that if you choose breast preservation for any breast cancer except LCIS, radiation is part of your primary treatment. So when you have an invasive breast cancer or DCIS, radiation *must* be part of your treatment if you selected a lumpectomy (see Decision Tree 6). Chemotherapy, like the other systemic therapies such as hormonal therapy and immunotherapy, is an *adjuvant* therapy in the treatment of breast cancer—an "add-on." This doesn't mean it isn't necessary. For breast cancers larger than one centimeter or, regardless of size, if even one axillary node is positive, chemotherapy is considered a *necessary* part of treatment. As a result of several major clinical trials, the chemotherapy that is most used precedes radiation. However, chemotherapy is not a substitute for radiotherapy. And radiation therapy is not a substitute for chemotherapy. *The two therapies are not interchangeable.* Current research is attempting to show that chemotherapy/hormonal therapy can substitute for radiation, but, thus far, clinical trials have not shown this to be the case.

Comprehensive, external beam radiation of the breast is regarded as the standard of care in breast preservation. "Why," you may ask, "is radiation added to the surgery? Why isn't a very wide excision enough? After all, the surgery removed the lump of cancer plus a rim of normal tissue. My surgeon even said, 'We got it all out.' Why do we need radiation?"

Clinical trials have showed that if there were no radiation following the lumpectomy, breast cancer would recur in the breast significantly more frequently than in breasts that were radiated following a lumpectomy. This finding suggests that, in addition to the tumor, individual breast cancer cells or tiny clusters of them—too small to be detected by mammography—are scattered throughout the breast. If not irradiated and thereby killed, they persist and eventually the breast cancer recurs. Or they can become an origination point for future metastases.

Numerous studies before 1980—first in Europe, later in the United States—showed that with progressively less surgery, radiation became an increasingly important component of treatment. It was as if the radiation took the place of the missing surgery.

It is evident from these studies that radiation is a necessary component of breast preservation. You may accept this fact intellectually but still dread having the treatment. Radiation of real people seems anathema. How can it be carried out safely? After all, isn't radiation harmful? Doesn't radiation *cause* cancer? Why do we use it to *treat* cancer?

Chapter 2, you may recall, deals with this issue. Yes, radiation in very low doses can cause cancer. Fortunately, the dose of radiation required to *eradicate* breast cancer cells is much higher than the dose of

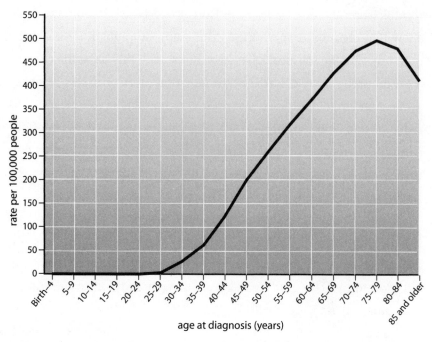

rate per 100,000 people

age at diagnosis (years)

Figure 11 The increase of breast cancer with age. Diagnosed breast cancer is much more frequent in elderly women.

radiation that *causes* cancer. The dose that kills breast cancer cells is known as a tumoricidal dose. For breast cancer cells, the tumoricidal dose is between 4,500 and 5,000 centigray (or 45–50 Gray) delivered relatively slowly. Moreover, breast cells are most susceptible to radiation when the breast tissue is developing—roughly between the ages of 13 and 30 years, far below the age of most women with breast cancer. The ages when women are most likely to get breast cancer are seen in Figure 11. Now do you see why radiation for breast cancer isn't likely to cause breast cancer? The treatment dose of radiation is too high, and the age of susceptible women is too low. So in the context of treatment, radiation isn't bad for you. In fact, in the context of treatment, radiation is helpful—if it is used effectively.

When you've gotten past that hurdle, you'll have other questions.

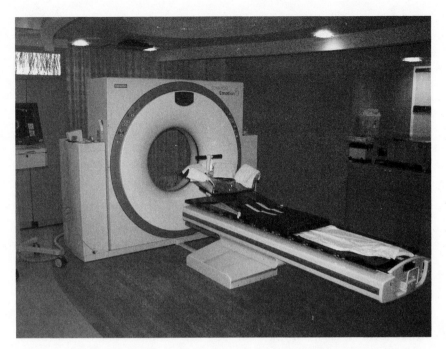

Figure 12 A CT simulator in which a CT scanner has been integrated into a standard simulator (which can also do the job). The low-energy x-rays produced by the simulator enable the radiation oncologist to take regular x-ray films that identify the target for treatment.

How soon after my surgery will my radiation therapy begin? How long will it continue? What will I experience? Will there be side effects? Aftereffects? How is radiation carried out? What happens to my breast after the initial treatments for breast preservation have been completed?

In the first step of radiation of the breast, you, the patient, are placed on a machine called a simulator, which plans the radiation that will be used in your treatment. The simulator can be combined with a CT scanner (Figure 12) to help localize the tumor bed. Think of a simulator as a machine with two functions: (1) it produces low-energy x-rays that enable the radiation oncologist to take standard x-ray pictures, and (2) it performs all the movements of a linear accelerator

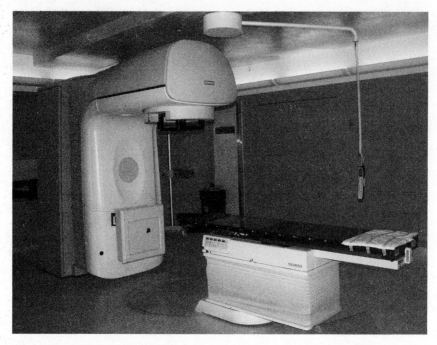

Figure 13 This treatment machine is a dual energy 1,800-electron volt linear accelerator capable of producing 6 million electron volts (6 MeV) and also 18 million electron volts (18 MeV). This high-energy unit can also produce electron *beams* ranging from 6 MeV to 18 MeV.

—the high-energy machine used to treat your breast cancer—and therefore it also can replicate the *treatment* movements of the linear accelerator.

By virtue of its high-energy beam, the linear accelerator (Figure 13) cannot take satisfactory x-ray pictures. Consequently, it cannot verify the area that it is to treat. The simulator, by virtue of its movement capability, allows the radiation oncologist to replicate the treatment, and to take x-rays that verify and localize the planned treatment. Think of a pilot simulating flight on a flight simulator; he or she doesn't take the plane up while learning to fly.

At the time of simulation, as part of the planning process, all necessary accessories are developed to keep the patient in position and localize the treatment area. These accessories are then used when the patient is on the linear accelerator. Tiny permanent marks (often called tattoos) may also be placed to help localize the treatment area. Laser beams also are used to help keep the patient in the correct position.

It is very important to note that while simulation is taking place, you are never alone. You are watched through a special leaded-glass window that protects the technologists and radiation oncologists watching you through the window. You can be heard, because microphones are in the simulation room and the speakers are in the outside planning room. If you call out, the planning process can be stopped immediately and your radiation simulator technologist and/or radiation oncologist will then enter the room to attend to your needs.

The scheduling of simulation involves both time on the simulator and availability of the radiation oncologist. Try to call for an appointment enough in advance after your surgery to give everyone plenty of lead time.

The simulator is used for all types of cancer, not just for breast cancer. What the cancers have in common is that a *target* must be established. The initial breast cancer target is the entire breast down to the chest wall (see Box 10). The area to be treated is larger than the target because it includes a small amount of normal tissue that surrounds the tumor bed. Thus, the *treatment* area for breast cancer encompasses the entire breast, the underlying chest wall, and a small bit of the lung under the chest wall.

The initial large treatment area of the breast is planned through opposed, tangential fields. A CT scan or ultrasound can help define the angle of the tangential fields, but it is not mandatory. The amount of lung that is to be included in the treatment area already is well documented by the low-energy x-ray films from the simulator.

Your radiation oncologist may mention the word "blocks" when

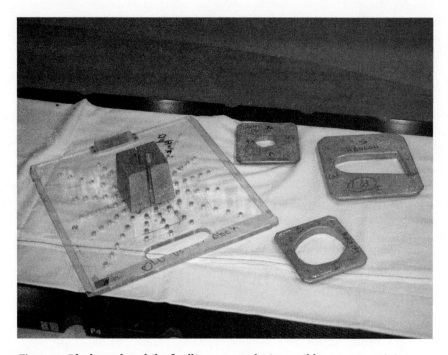

Figure 14 Blocks and multileaf collimators make it possible to treat a minimum of uninvolved tissue. Often, blocks are used to protect normal, contiguous tissue from the high-energy beam of the linear accelerator. These blocks, specially designed by the radiation oncologist when planning the treatment, are made from a lead-like alloy that does not weigh as much as lead. Multileaf collimators can replace blocks and perform the same function.

describing your proposed radiation treatment (Figure 14). Planned by the radiation oncologist at the time of simulation, blocks prevent the radiation beam from reaching contiguous normal tissues. New linear accelerators have multileaf collimators. When these are in position, they eliminate the necessity for blocks. The leaves of the collimators essentially *are* blocks, and they also shape the area to be treated. Whether blocks or multileaf collimators are used, the result will be the same— a shaped field that will block the radiation beam from affecting contiguous normal tissue.

Box 10 Limited Field Radiation Using a Linear
Accelerator

Like their surgical colleagues, radiation oncologists are
attempting to do less rather than more. They are examining
whether it is necessary to irradiate the *whole* breast with external beam radiation after lumpectomy. Studies are being con-
ducted on carefully selected patients to see if a field smaller
than the entire breast will suffice. A clinical trial has been initiated to test whether limited external beam radiation will give
the same survival and recurrence results as whole breast irradiation. The results will not be known for many years—too
late, unfortunately, for patients who right now want the assur-
ance of effective treatment with a limited field.

If the axillary lymph nodes are to be treated in addition to the
breast, the lymph node area is treated by a single, shaped field. This
lymph node field is aimed from the front of the patient and is planned
to be shallow; it penetrates only to the depth of the lymph nodes. If it
is necessary to bring the final dose to the center of the axilla, a small
"boost" beam is simulated to be aimed from behind the patient.

A boost is a higher, tumoricidal (cancer-killing) dose of radiation
administered to a very small field: *the tumor bed plus a margin.* In this
way the patient avoids the side effects that would occur if the entire
area were given this higher dose. (For example, if the entire breast was
treated with a tumoricidal dose, unfortunate side effects would result.)

Clearly, this kind of radiation treatment is extremely complex and requires sophisticated equipment. It should be performed by a skilled radiation oncologist who has an entire team of physicists, dosimetrists, and radiation technologists to provide the needed technical support. Sophisticated equipment and appropriate technical support minimize the chance of complications later. I have often said that if high-quality radiation is not available to a patient who lives in a remote area, it is better to have a mastectomy than to suffer the unfortunate aftereffects of poorly performed radiation.

Radiation oncologists are basically "techies"—devotees of the newest and best equipment. Manufacturers of radiation equipment are sensitive to this fact. Thus, new concepts are continually being incorporated into advanced equipment, benefiting patients, radiation oncologists, and technical staff alike. For example, we have seen that CT scanners have been introduced into the simulation process. This means that, instead of obtaining a separate CT, planning can take place directly on the CT simulator, thereby speeding up the entire process for both the patient and the radiation therapy staff. In addition, multileaf collimators are almost routinely being used on linear accelerators in large facilities. Dynamic treatment is being perfected: not only do the leaves of the beam-shaping collimators move, but the couch also moves, making the shaped beam even more complex. These dramatic changes require physicians and staff alike to have special training so that they qualify to handle such highly developed equipment.

Besides the radiation oncologist, two specially trained professionals whom you may never see—the dosimetrist and the radiation physicist—are involved in planning your treatment. In addition, when special blocks are used, a trained radiation technologist must prepare them. The dosimetrist generates a computerized plan from the contour of the breast and the simulated fields. The radiation physicist oversees the computerization and is available for consultation in the general planning. The computerized plan generated by the dosimetrist is the basis for the calculated dose to each field. The computerized plan and the dose must be checked by the radiation oncology physician in charge *before any treatment is initiated.*

Thus, considerable activity takes place before you are actually treated on the linear accelerator. Your treatment usually does not begin for at least two to three working days after the simulation. Of course, it goes without saying that any emergency takes precedence. Day or night, your radiation oncologist can, and often does, carry out all the steps necessary to treat you in a crisis.

So that you won't worry about the unknown, at the time of simulation you should be shown the linear accelerator that will treat you. As with the simulator, you are not isolated in the linear accelerator room. Microphones will capture your every word, and at least two television cameras are trained on you. *You really are in control.* You need only ask and the treatment will be stopped, to be resumed whenever you are ready. If you cannot speak, a prearranged signal, such as lifting a finger or hand, is enough to halt the process.

Typically, treatment on the linear accelerator takes place every day, usually at the same time. You are put in position by the radiation technologist. Laser light beams directed at you, plus any accessories your radiation oncologist devised at the time of simulation, ensure that you are in the same position each time you are treated. Verification films from these high-energy machines are taken on the linear accelerator on a routine basis and approved or changed by your radiation oncology physician (after comparison with the approved simulation films). You are carefully observed daily by your radiation oncology technologist and by your radiation oncology nurse. Any deviation is reported to your radiation oncologist, who examines you at least once a week.

That is the customary routine. Obviously, any deviation will take you out of the routine. Your radiation oncologist will supervise your care and will be the primary physician in charge of your case while you are being irradiated. Once treatment has concluded, he or she will arrange your follow-up appointments. Since the radiation oncologist is part of your treatment team, this individual will keep the other members of your treatment team fully informed.

Brachytherapy and Limited Field Therapy

Brachytherapy is an old modality that has been rediscovered. Today, thin plastic tubes containing radioactive seeds, or balloons containing a single intensely radioactive seed, are surgically placed in the tumor bed, generally at the time of the lumpectomy. In the past, low-dose-rate seeds were placed in thin plastic tubes known as catheters. When treating breast cancer, the catheters were surgically inserted by the radiation oncologist into the tumor bed of the breast. This form of brachytherapy was used as a boost. Generally, it took about forty-eight hours to deliver the planned dose of radiation to the tumor bed.

The initial results of a brachytherapy boost were beautiful. But after five years or so, the area of the brachytherapy boost frequently became very hard, dense, and fibrotic, making it difficult to examine the patient's breast. This late complication precluded the use of low-dose-rate brachytherapy. When electrons became available, they were used instead. The long-term side effects of electron boosts were negligible compared to the long-term side effects of the low-dose-rate brachytherapy boosts.

Today brachytherapy of the breast is carried out with *high-dose-rate* seeds. The overall time of treatment is considerably shorter.

As a result, brachytherapy is having another heyday. It is being used in several different ways and with different end points.

One approach is the "mammosite" treatment, which has been given a great deal of press. A balloon containing an extremely hot radioactive seed is surgically placed in the tumor bed at the time of the lumpectomy. By this means, radiation is delivered to the tumor bed. The mammosite treatment lasts a relatively short time because the seed is so intensely radioactive. The balloon conforms to the tumor bed. The issue of whether an adequate, homogeneous dose of radiation is delivered by the mammosite approach is debated vociferously by radiotherapists. Only time and recurrence rates will give the answer.

The long-term complications of using high-dose-rate brachytherapy alone are also being explored. In this scenario, only brachytherapy is used to treat the breast—not any external beam radiation such as that which comes from a linear accelerator. The advantage is that the treatment time is very short. The potential disadvantage is that the complication rate is unknown—especially over the long term. It is recommended that this approach be reserved for older women with a potentially short life span who require prompt treatment.

Side Effects

Radiation can have two types of side effects—acute (or short term) and long term. Both are dependent on the site being treated. It is the side effects of breast irradiation that interest us at this time.

Short-Term Effects

The acute side effects of breast irradiation are those that occur during treatment of breast cancer with radiation. As radiation proceeds, your skin will become progressively pink, then red—just like a sunburn. Once radiation has been completed, your skin will tan and even undergo dry peeling, as it does when you have a sunburn. Your nipples may become very sensitive to any clothing that rubs against them. You are cautioned not to use creams on the treated area and to forgo wearing a bra. Instead, you are encouraged to wear a satiny, silky camisole that doesn't have front seams. Some women benefit from rubbing the liquid that oozes from the cut leaves of the aloe vera plant over the surface of their breasts during radiation treatment.

Women who are not obese and who have bra size AA to B generally sail through radiation treatments. Women with a size DD cup and large, pendulous breasts may have trouble. They may develop "moist desquamation" in the fold under the breast. Although this denuded area under a pendulous breast can be very painful (it almost never becomes infected), the condition is not life threatening, and the pain may be relieved by placing cotton soaked in a boric acid solution in the area. Occasionally a woman becomes so uncomfortable from the moist, denuded skin under her breast that she must lie down most of the time when she is not being treated, thereby exposing the underside of her breast to the air or to a fan.

Another acute side effect that occurs during radiation treatments is fatigue. It is not evident why this is so. Radiation for breast preservation does not treat your internal organs. Only your breast and, in some cases, your draining lymph nodes are treated. All these are structures outside the main part of your body. Perhaps the daily trips to the radiation facility for approximately six weeks play a role. Regardless of the cause, the fatigue is usually not very troublesome. It disappears after the radiation has been completed.

You may have heard that you should expect other acute side effects, such as alteration of your blood count, loss of hair, diarrhea, nausea, and vomiting. These misconceptions are common.

Relatively little bone marrow is in the treatment field for breast cancer, so you should not expect a significant alteration of your blood counts as a result of radiation. Many women, however, have had chemotherapy prior to their radiation, at which time their blood count was monitored carefully and frequently. (Chemotherapy is systemic therapy and will affect bone marrow throughout the body. The number of cells derived from bone marrow—white blood cells, red blood cells, and platelets—often decreases significantly during chemotherapy.) Radiation after chemotherapy will not begin until your blood count is normal. Radiation oncologists take one blood count before, one during, and one at the end of radiation. There is no need to check more frequently.

What about hair loss, diarrhea, nausea, and vomiting? Remember that the side effects of radiation are specific to the site being treated. This means that if other parts of the body were treated, other side effects would take place. Since only your breast and possibly the draining lymph node areas are treated, you should not have symptoms of diarrhea, nausea, vomiting, and hair loss. In breast irradiation your scalp, your abdomen, your pelvis, and your stomach are not treated. If you have problems of diarrhea, nausea, vomiting, or hair loss, look for another cause.

Certainly, you will *not* be radioactive after your treatment with the linear accelerator. You and your sexual partner need have no worries on that account.

Each radiation oncologist has a bag of tricks to deal with the short-term, temporary side effects of radiation. However, the most important trick is patience. You should know that all acute side effects are temporary and will be gone soon after the radiation has been completed. Only the memory will linger.

Long-Term Effects

What about long-term side effects?

What does the breast look like and feel like long after it has been irradiated with external beam irradiation? Well, your treated breast may look *slightly* tanner than the untreated breast. Perhaps it may feel a bit rubbery. (The rubbery feel is not apt to be apprehended by anyone except the patient, her significant other, and the radiation oncologist who has been trained to look for it.) These are the usual side effects of radiation to the breast. Both are very mild long-term aftereffects.

One possible side effect that is particularly bothersome is lymph-edema, or swelling, of the arm on the side of the affected breast. You may know that the incidence of arm edema was reduced when radical mastectomies were replaced by modified radical mastectomies and further reduced when modified radical mastectomies were replaced by breast preservation. Postoperative radiation usually was not given to these women. This trend suggests that all or part of the arm swelling is caused by the extensiveness of the surgery in the axilla. We now know this to be the case. However, the fact that the number of cases of arm lymphedema has significantly declined is of no comfort to the woman who suffers from it. It is a side effect she wishes she could avoid.

Lymphedema of the arm is frequently noted *after* the radiation for breast preservation has been completed. That is why radiation has been cited as the sole cause of arm edema. However, it can be found in women who have had a mastectomy without radiation. When it oc-curs after breast preservation, it is generally associated with the *com-bination* of surgery and radiation, a result of vigorous surgical dissec-tion of the axilla in addition to radiation of the axilla.

Women who require both a mastectomy and radiation should be aware of the possible long-term radiation complications that may ensue if reconstruction is carried out. Many women opt to have im-mediate reconstruction—placement of the implant at the time of the mastectomy—thinking that it will save them a second surgery. The problem is that radiation of the implant, when necessary, can have the unwanted side effect of "capsular contraction." To you, the pa-tient, the implant becomes progressively harder and smaller than it was originally. Such capsular contraction often is striking enough to be seen on serial mammograms. Occasionally, it is sufficiently severe and uncomfortable that the implant must be removed. Discuss this side effect with your radiation oncologist as well as with your plastic surgeon when you plan your reconstruction. The obvious way to avoid the problem is to have the implant placed after the radiation has been completed. Even then, capsular contraction can occur, presumably because the surgical bed induces it.

Another surgical way to avoid the problem of capsular contraction is with a TRAM flap, in which a breast mound is constructed from the woman's own abdominal tissue. It is a major procedure and should be discussed in detail with the plastic surgeon at the time reconstruction options are being considered.

Although a TRAM flap appears to be the ideal solution following a mastectomy, the radiation oncologist will find it impossible to know where to place the radiation boost if the TRAM flap is carried out *before* the radiation. That is why the TRAM flap is best carried out afterward. It does mean a second surgery, and some inexperienced plastic surgeons prefer not to operate on radiated tissue, stating incorrectly that the radiation inhibits healing.

Other side effects of radiation are rare, but should be mentioned. Occasionally a patient develops a dry, hacking cough. If a chest x-ray is obtained, it may show a haziness in the part of the lung that was treated. This is called radiation pneumonitis and can be thought of as an inflammation of the lung. It generally is not associated with fever and is self-limiting. Steroids, such as prednisone, can be prescribed, and the radiation pneumonitis promptly vanishes. Generally, it is not necessary to prescribe anything, including steroids. The problem simply disappears by itself.

Very rarely (I have seen it in two cases out of the thousands I have treated) a woman will develop hardening and redness of the treated breast. Although a complete workup shows that it is *not* recurrent cancer, the cause of this fibrosis is unknown. In the two cases that I saw, the radiation dose was reviewed and proved to be correct; no nonradiation causes were obvious. A biopsy of the breast did not show any background abnormalities. Thus, fibrosis can occur—albeit extremely rarely—without apparent cause.

Other rare long-term complications include subtle skin changes such as telangectasias (the appearance of spidery blood vessels on the previously irradiated skin surface); damage to bone (rib fractures), muscles, or nerves; and the unusual possibility of second cancers caused by radiation many years after the radiation is completed. Most of these complications are dose related and are avoided by well-trained radiation oncologists. Many informed consent forms (which should be signed by the patient before any radiation is administered) refer to these potential complications. By their nature, informed consents give the worst possible scenarios, which fortunately are exceedingly rare.

Remember . . .

- If you have a lumpectomy, radiation in addition to the surgery is part of the primary treatment for breast preservation.
- Radiation and chemotherapy are not alternatives in the treatment of breast cancer. Frequently both are necessary.
- *Planning* of treatment with radiation is carried out with a simulator, which replicates all of the movements of the linear accelerator without treating the patient.
- *Treatment* of breast cancer is usually carried out with a linear accelerator. However, brachytherapy is once again being used.
- Since the simulator uses low-energy x-rays and the linear accelerator uses high-energy x-rays, the pictures taken by the two are very different.
- Side effects of radiation include reddening of the skin during breast preservation treatments, some peeling of the skin when radiation is over, and a slight rubbery feel to the breast long after treatment is finished.

- Side effects you will *not* have when treated for breast cancer after a lumpectomy include hair loss, decreased blood count, diarrhea, nausea, and vomiting.
- If you have had reconstruction and require radiation, capsular contractures are side effects that you should discuss with your radiation oncologist and your plastic surgeon.

Chapter 8   Systemic Therapy

Systemic therapy treats the whole body. It is delivered by the medical oncologist member of your treatment team. It is given to combat metastases—the spread of cancer cells from the primary tumor in your breast to other sites. It can also be used to inhibit the growth of an existing cancer, even to shrink it. Chemotherapy, hormonal therapy, and biological therapy are the three forms of systemic treatment, all of which can be given as pills or by injection. The therapy gets into your bloodstream, going everywhere and acting everywhere. It gets into your entire system—hence the term *systemic*. Chemotherapy is the form most people know, but hormonal therapy has become increasingly important in the last several years. Biological therapy, which primarily includes antibodies, has raised high hopes.

Systemic therapy is not interchangeable with surgery or radiation. Both surgery and radiation are *local* treatments and therefore are used for localized disease, such as the tumor in your breast or lymph nodes.

Decision Tree 7 Systemic Therapy

Phase 1

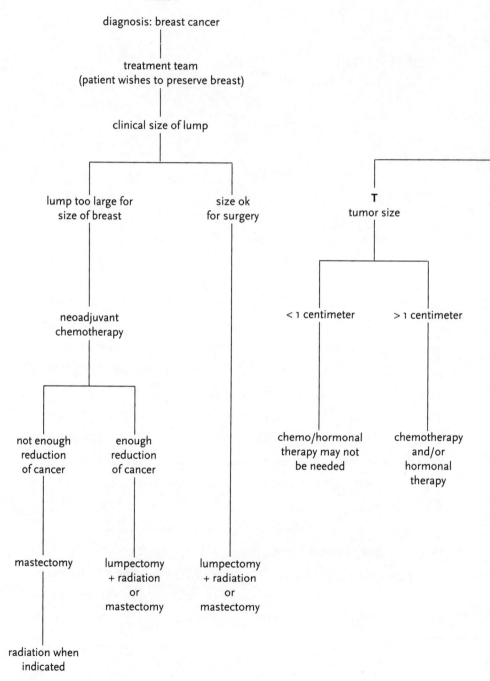

diagnosis: breast cancer

treatment team
(patient wishes to preserve breast)

clinical size of lump

lump too large for
size of breast

size ok
for surgery

T
tumor size

neoadjuvant
chemotherapy

< 1 centimeter

> 1 centimeter

not enough
reduction
of cancer

enough
reduction
of cancer

chemo/hormonal
therapy may not
be needed

chemotherapy
and/or
hormonal
therapy

mastectomy

lumpectomy
+ radiation
or
mastectomy

lumpectomy
+ radiation
or
mastectomy

radiation when
indicated

Phase 2

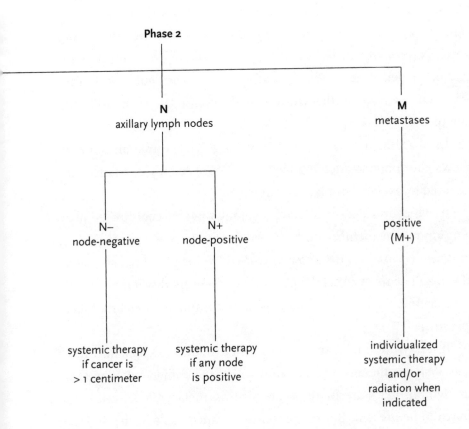

N
axillary lymph nodes

M
metastases

N–
node-negative

N+
node-positive

positive
(M+)

systemic therapy
if cancer is
> 1 centimeter

systemic therapy
if any node
is positive

individualized
systemic therapy
and/or
radiation when
indicated

Only systemic therapy can combat cancer cells that might be lurking elsewhere in your body.

Decision Tree 7 shows that systemic therapy can be used during two different phases of your treatment: Phase 1, before the staging of your cancer ("neoadjuvant"); phase 2, after pathologic staging ("adjuvant"). In phase 1 you would like to preserve your breast. You haven't had surgery yet. Your pathological stage is unknown, although your clinical stage can be assumed from your physical examination. Your tumor is too large for the size of your breast; therefore, a lumpectomy cannot be performed without inviting a poor cosmetic result. Your treatment team agrees that you are an ideal candidate for neoadjuvant therapy.

In phase 2, you have already had surgery. The tree on the right shows your options after you have had a lumpectomy or mastectomy followed by axillary lymph node surgery.

In whichever phase you have systemic therapy, coordinated planning among the members of your treatment team is essential *before any treatment begins*. You need to be involved in this planning, so that all of you will be ready to set the plan in motion or modify it if necessary.

Systemic therapy after staging is more common, so let's start there (phase 2).

If the lymph nodes under your arm are found to contain cancer cells, systemic therapy most certainly will be recommended. When axillary lymph nodes are found to be positive, metastatic disease is not *proven* to be present. But the presence of cancer cells in the draining axillary lymph nodes makes it clear that cancer cells have left the primary site in your breast, and it is *presumed* that they have gone beyond the lymph nodes into the rest of the body. In other words, your cancer could be metastatic.

When systemic therapy is used to treat presumed disease, it is called *adjuvant therapy*. The word "adjuvant" in this context means "add-on." Numerous studies have found that adjuvant chemotherapy or adjuvant hormonal therapy reduces the number of expected metastases. If your breast cancer is more than one centimeter in diameter and/or if your axillary lymph nodes are shown by the pathologist to contain breast cancer cells, expect to be offered adjuvant chemotherapy or adjuvant hormonal therapy in addition to your primary local treatments of surgery and radiation.

When the cancer is large or when the cancer is metastatic—in other words, beyond an early stage—systemic chemotherapy or hormonal therapy can be used as an adjuvant or as primary treatment to treat breast cancer directly.

The kind of adjuvant chemotherapy or adjuvant hormonal therapy that will be offered depends on several factors that your medical oncologist takes into account before making a recommendation. These factors include your age, your menopausal status, whether or not your breast cancer cells contain certain hormone receptors—many factors.

Although the statistical benefit of adjuvant chemotherapy to women with early-stage breast cancer is very small, it is now routine to offer chemotherapy or hormonal therapy to all women with breast cancer who have had a lumpectomy, positive axillary nodes, or cancers larger than one centimeter, regardless of their lymph node status. Systemic therapy is offered to eliminate *potential* metastases. Most women elect to have the "most aggressive" treatment in order to give themselves the best chance for potential cure. For most women, even a very small statistical advantage is worth temporarily compromising their quality of life. Premenopausal women generally wish to have adjuvant chemotherapy. A small statistical gain is better than no gain. And remember, you are not a statistic. Similarly, postmenopausal women, when offered hormonal therapy (they often are offered chemotherapy), tend to select what they are offered.

Depending on the size of your cancer, you might have systemic therapy at an earlier phase of your treatment—before you have breast surgery and before your cancer is pathologically staged (see phase 1 of Decision Tree 7).

Suppose you've had a needle biopsy or small incisional biopsy, and invasive breast cancer has been diagnosed. You want to preserve your breast if you can, but you don't know if a lumpectomy is possible. That is because your tumor is so large in relation to the size of your breast—a five-centimeter lump, let's say, in your bra-size-A breast —that a lumpectomy would deform the breast. Your physician may recommend neoadjuvant chemotherapy to reduce the size of the tumor. If the tumor can be shrunk sufficiently—in this example, to a one- to two-centimeter tumor in a size A bra—you will be eligible for breast preservation with lumpectomy and radiation. If you turn out *not* to be eligible, then breast preservation will not be possible and you will need to have a mastectomy.

You have already seen your surgeon, but if you are a candidate for neoadjuvant chemotherapy, your first treating physician will be your medical oncologist. (Your treatment team determines whether you are a candidate for this treatment.) Before neoadjuvant therapy you will be sent to your radiation oncologist to have little permanent marks (often called tattoos) placed on your breast to define the original size of the primary cancer in order to plan the radiation boost to be administered after your surgery. Not all radiation oncologists feel a boost is necessary for stage I and stage II breast cancers that have been treated with breast preservation techniques. But all agree that a large breast cancer requires a boost, even a large cancer that has been reduced in size by neoadjuvant therapy.

Now you are ready for systemic therapy. New and classic chemotherapeutic agents such as taxol, adriamycin, and cytoxan (singly and in various combinations) are being tested in a variety of clinical trials. The timing of these agents is also being tested. Hormonal agents, including the aromatase inhibitors, are also being tried. Studies combining biologic agents with chemotherapy (for example, herceptin with either a taxane or cisplatin) are under way as well.

As you can see from Decision Tree 7, phase i, if the cancer is not sufficiently reduced in size by the neoadjuvant therapy, you should have a mastectomy. If the tumor shrinks sufficiently, you will be eligible for breast preservation with a lumpectomy and radiation. I'll say more momentarily about the coordination of systemic therapy with radiation therapy.

Following the definitive surgery, whether lumpectomy and staging axillary dissection or modified radical mastectomy (which includes an axillary dissection), the surgical-pathologic staging of your breast cancer is carried out. Based on that stage, you may receive chemo- or hormonal therapy.

If the cancer in your breast is of a size that is one centimeter or less, you will need radiation in addition to the lumpectomy, *but not chemo-/hormonal therapy*. If cancer is found in any lymph node under the arm, chemo- and/or hormonal therapy will be recommended. If you have metastases, your metastatic status will determine the type of therapy to be offered.

Chemotherapy

Chemotherapy consists of "cytotoxic" drugs, which kill cells by virtue of their toxicity. Unfortunately, chemotherapeutic agents are not very discriminating; they affect both cancer cells and normal cells. Hence, they trigger a multitude of side effects that result predominantly from their effect on normal cells.

Well-known examples of chemotherapeutic agents are adriamycin (also known as doxorubicin), cytoxan (also known as cyclophosphamide), and the taxanes such as taxol (paclitaxel) and taxotere (doxataxel), to name a few.

Chemotherapeutic drugs are generally used as combinations. Therefore, their side effects are usually added together. Combination chemotherapy used in early-stage breast cancer is *adjuvant* chemotherapy and has an entirely different impact from chemotherapy or hormonal therapy used in a nonadjuvant (primary) setting.

Doctors use the terms "complete" and "partial" when discussing the response of a cancer to chemotherapy. A complete response is a full 100 percent response. A partial response is, by definition, a 50 percent response. But it is the durability of the response that is important. It doesn't help you to have a fleeting complete response. You need that response to last a long time.

The durability of the response is not regarded as significant in neoadjuvant therapy. If the tumor is sufficiently reduced in size, it will be surgically removed by a lumpectomy. So only a partial response is necessary, because that response is followed by a lumpectomy and radiation. With an appropriate radiation boost, one that takes into account the size of the original tumor, the response should be durable. Only time will tell if this is indeed the case.

Women who have not yet undergone menopause (generally 50 years of age or younger) are the ones routinely offered chemotherapy as first-line treatment, as opposed to hormonal therapy. Although in the past two forms of combination chemotherapy were offered to women who were to receive chemotherapy, today the adriamycin-containing regimen is customarily offered in the form of adriamycin and cytoxan (AC), to which taxol often is added.

The other form of combination chemotherapy was known as CMF, which is the acronym for cytoxan, methotrexate, and 5-fluorouracil. The adriamycin-containing regimen ultimately became more favored on the part of both medical oncologists and patients and today is the regimen most often recommended. The reason is twofold: it is the shorter regimen (four cycles as opposed to six cycles), and it is believed to be the more aggressive of the two regimens because the side effects are more severe. Many women prefer a shorter period of treatment because every day seems like an eternity when you are experiencing the side effects of chemotherapy.

After CMF fell into disrepute, the methotrexate was replaced by adriamycin. The acronym is now CAF. This is the basic combination chemotherapy delivered in many institutions. Other drugs, like taxol, may be added to the CAF. Also, many institutions are using chemotherapy more frequently. Instead of every three weeks, the chemotherapy is given every two weeks. These are permutations on a single theme, but the timing of chemotherapy may turn out to be of major importance. Only carefully planned clinical trials will give us the answer.

The issue of how to interweave radiation and chemotherapy has been debated by radiation and medical oncologists since the time chemotherapy was first recommended as an adjuvant in the treatment of breast cancer. After all, it is argued, radiation is part of the *primary* treatment for women who have had breast preservation, and chemotherapy is an adjuvant. Is it more important to combat residual microscopic disease in the breast, which may serve as a nidus for a recurrence in the breast as well as for distant metastases (local disease), or is it more important to treat presumed metastatic disease? Should all the primary treatment be completed first, before embarking on adjuvant treatment? At this time, there is no accepted answer to these questions.

Medical oncologists can help deal with the side effects of chemotherapy, which can be as severe emotionally as physically. This is a powerful reason to select your medical oncologist carefully. He or she should be not only well trained, but also understanding of you and your loved ones. Most important, your medical oncologist should be empathetic to *you*.

There is one side effect that everyone knows about. You will lose your hair with most chemotherapy drugs. But it will grow back once you no longer undergo chemotherapy. Patients have various approaches to hair loss. Women (and also men) are very attached to their hair . . . they don't want to lose it. If they do lose it, what then? Yes, there are wigs, but they are not considered de rigeur by all.

I had a memorable young woman patient several years ago, a beautiful model who had exquisite red hair prior to treatment. Of course she lost her hair, but she never wore a wig. Instead, she wore scarves and wide-brimmed hats and looked incredibly glamorous throughout her treatment. She taught all our women patients how to wear scarves and hats. She even instructed our nurses, so that they could teach other patients. Further, she taught patients and nurses how to use cosmetics and how to dress. Needless to say, she had quite an impact on all our patients, men included. Unhappily, she lost more than her hair; her husband left her when her hair did. When she completed treatment, it grew back as before, a lustrous, beautiful red. When her hair returned, so did her husband. Remarkably, she took him back.

This young woman spent her time and energy helping others to improve their self-image. She had an impact on them that was priceless. She really cared, and each individual she touched knew it.

More mundanely, I learned from her that wigs weren't necessary for all who had lost their hair. "Wigs are too expensive, too warm, too uncomfortable in general," patients complained. Many found other nonwig solutions. Baseball hats could be used—some bejeweled, sequined, and elegant for formal wear, others casual and stylish. One patient claimed she had about two hundred baseball hats by the time her chemotherapy was over. She never wore a wig and looked wonderful throughout.

Still others experimented with different colors and styles of wigs, achieving images vastly different from their prechemotherapy days.

Did you ever want to be a redhead? Get a red wig. Want to be a long-haired blonde? Get a long-haired blonde wig. Get several cheap wigs from your local department store and have fun with them! Chemotherapy need not be a disaster. Even after chemotherapy is behind you, wigs can counteract a bad hair day. Women who have never had chemotherapy can use wigs to cover up uncooperative hairdos.

Then there are those who don't do anything to cover up this side effect. They go out in public with their cool, chemotherapy-bald heads. They tend to be women with long, swan-like necks and wonderfully shaped skulls, who wear big, important earrings and feel perfectly comfortable with their bald look.

Some who do not like to show baldness when out in public recognize, when their hair begins to grow back and is one to two inches long, that they look marvelous that way; they wear that look for a very long time.

Hormonal Therapy

Hormonal therapy for breast cancer uses a class of substances known as antiestrogens. This makes sense, because it is acknowledged that one particular estrogen is involved in the promotion of breast cancer.

Adjuvant hormonal therapy for breast cancer is generally offered to postmenopausal women who have a rich supply of estrogen receptors in their breast cancer cells. These women are known as having estrogen-receptor-positive breast cancer. Your pathology report will indicate whether you are ER positive or negative. If you are postmenopausal and ER negative, you may be offered chemotherapy by your medical oncologist.

The best-known of the antiestrogens is tamoxifen, or nolvadex (Box 11). It has been around a long time and has a proven record in

Box 11 Tamoxifen

At this writing, hundreds of thousands of women have used tamoxifen. They have been followed in clinical trials worldwide for ten to fifteen years or longer. The positive and negative effects of tamoxifen have been well established and extensively published in the medical literature. As a result, the medical community is very familiar with tamoxifen.

Tamoxifen started life many years ago as a contraceptive. When it was clear that it failed in this task—women became pregnant while on tamoxifen—it was taken off the shelf. Fifteen years later, it came back to life as an antiestrogen in the fight against breast cancer.

One of the most useful drugs available, tamoxifen was highly effective in combating advanced breast cancer, and its side effects, compared to those of chemotherapy, were relatively mild. Because of its antiestrogen effects, it was not used in premenopausal women.

After many years of successful use of tamoxifen in treating advanced breast cancer, the National Cancer Institute recommended that it be used as an adjuvant to treat the huge numbers of postmenopausal, estrogen-receptor-positive women with *early*-stage breast cancer.

Later, in the first breast cancer prevention trial, tamoxifen was found to prevent breast cancer in approximately 50 percent of women who had never had breast cancer but were considered to have a high risk for developing it. Tamoxifen was the first "chemopreventive" drug to be used against breast cancer.

treating both late-stage and early-stage cancer and, more recently, to "prevent" breast cancer.

Thus, tamoxifen plays various roles with respect to breast cancer. It is used to *treat* advanced breast cancer, it is used as an *adjuvant* for postmenopausal women with ER-positive breast cancer, and now it can be used to *prevent* breast cancer in high-risk women.

Despite its beneficial effects, tamoxifen does have two major drawbacks: (1) it has been found to have dual properties—that is, it functions not only as an antiestrogen but also as an estrogen; (2) its use is restricted to women whose breast cancer cells are found to have estrogen (and progesterone) receptors.

The second drawback has been handled expeditiously for many years. A simple laboratory test for estrogen and progesterone receptors is routinely carried out on all women with breast cancer. The results are available in your pathology report.

The first drawback is more complex. Tamoxifen functions primarily as an antiestrogen when used to combat breast cancer. However, published studies found that it also acts like an estrogen, causing such estrogen-related side effects as cancer of the breast and uterus. This property was evaluated very carefully in the first chemoprevention trial, where tamoxifen was used as a "chemopreventive" agent in 13,388 women who did not have a history of breast cancer but were considered to be at high risk for developing it.

I put the term "chemopreventive" in quotation marks because the Food and Drug Administration called tamoxifen a "risk-reducing agent" instead of a chemopreventive agent, based on the results of that trial: after six years, the 13,388 high-risk women had a startling 40–50 percent reduction in the expected number of invasive and noninvasive breast cancers.

In spite of these remarkable results, the press concentrated on the estrogen-like properties of tamoxifen. Since estrogen can cause breast

and uterine cancers (both in a very low incidence), tamoxifen was regarded with a great deal of suspicion by many. These reservations were
published in the medical literature and the popular media had a field
day. Women everywhere were confused and frightened.

The result of this bad press is best exemplified by my 65-year-old
patient with advanced metastatic breast cancer. This woman's medical
oncologist correctly recommended that she take tamoxifen to combat
her raging breast cancer. The woman refused to take the tamoxifen,
stating that she had read several articles in her local newspaper and
in national magazines which said that tamoxifen could cause cancer
of the uterus. And she did not want to die from cancer of the uterus!
Instead, she died of metastatic breast cancer. This poorly informed
woman was trading a potentially curable cancer for a lethal one.

Yes, it is true that tamoxifen can cause cancer of the uterus, but,
as the chemoprevention trial with tamoxifen confirmed, all 36 women
(of the 13,388 women in the six-year trial) who developed cancer of the
uterus had an early-stage cancer of the uterus, stage I, and had a low-
grade cancer. *They could be cured by hysterectomy alone.* One merely had
to read the results of the trial to know the true facts.

A second chemoprevention trial, the STAR trial, compares raloxifene with tamoxifen to see if they are equally effective in reducing
the expected number of cases of invasive and noninvasive breast cancer in 22,000 postmenopausal, high-risk women. Raloxifene, another
antiestrogen related to tamoxifen, appears to lack the estrogenic properties of tamoxifen and therefore may not cause any uterine cancer.
In this respect and others, raloxifene may well be superior to tamoxifen, but it does not have the long track record of tamoxifen and its
side effects are not as well known.

The relatively new class of antiestrogens known as *aromatase inhibitors* are generating high anticipation in the treatment of breast cancer. They are not antiestrogens per se; they interfere with the metabo-

lism of estrogen, thereby inactivating it and making it appear that estrogen was never present. The third or more generation of aromatase inhibitors is now being tested.

Thus, drugs like tamoxifen work against estrogen that is already present. Drugs like aromatase inhibitors work to prevent estrogen from developing. Although the end result is the same, the aromatase inhibitors theoretically should give an advantage because they do not allow estrogen to be produced. Clinical trials are currently under way to determine which drugs are superior.

Tamoxifen is still the standard against which all other endocrine manipulations of breast cancer must be measured. Raloxifene, the newer aromatase inhibitors, and other antiestrogens are being tested intensively to see whether any can replace, or perhaps be superior to, tamoxifen. Thus far, it seems that some third-generation aromatase inhibitors may surpass tamoxifen.

Biologic Therapy

Recently, a great deal of attention has focused on a class of agents known as targeted biologics. This form of systemic therapy is not yet part of the standard armamentarium of medical oncologists, but it is becoming increasingly important.

Targeted biologics are agents "targeted" against specific molecules or cancer cell components. They often have a cancer cell killer molecule attached, such as a molecule that delivers radiation or an active component of a chemotherapy drug. One of the reasons biologic agents are attractive is that they treat only the tissues against which they are targeted, bypassing normal, healthy tissues. They do not have the nasty side effects of chemotherapy, which unfortunately treats normal, healthy tissues as well as the cancer itself. Thus, the hateful consequences of chemotherapy (nausea, vomiting, hair loss) are not prominent side effects of these targeted biologic agents.

The best-known of these targeting agents are antibodies produced in the immune response. Immunology includes the study of antibodies. Although it is a very old field, recent developments are making immunology one of the fastest-moving areas of biologic research.

Cancer vaccines and antibodies against newly formed blood vessels that cancers promote (thereby enabling them to obtain blood-borne nutrients)—all are among the rubric of targeted biologic agents. These are general antibodies, agents targeted against various components of cancer cells or blood vessels, which have general significance. There are also agents targeted against breast cancer specifically. Herceptin, for instance, is an antibody targeted against certain breast cancer cells that have HER-2 neu receptors. Thus herceptin is potentially a primary treatment for breast cancer. Currently it is being used against already established breast cancer—against recurrent local disease or metastatic breast cancer. Trials are under way to show that herceptin can be used against early-stage breast cancer. The targeted agents are limited in two ways: (1) they are effective only against HER-2 neu receptor positive cells, and (2) they seem to work best when given with certain chemotherapeutic drugs. As of this writing, a second generation of herceptin agents has generated a great deal of excitement and will most certainly induce further interest if and when the agents are approved by the FDA.

We are likely to hear much more about the newer targeted biological agents and their next generations as time goes on. In any increment of time, newer beneficial agents may become available to you.

Remember . . .

- Systemic therapy is not interchangeable with surgery or radiation which are local treatments for local disease. Systemic therapy treats the whole body.
- If your tumor is too large relative to your breast, preventing you

from preserving your breast with lumpectomy and radiation, you may be a candidate for neoadjuvant chemotherapy. This treatment, carried out before definitive treatment, is undertaken to reduce the tumor in your breast to a size where lumpectomy can be carried out without significantly deforming the breast.

- Neoadjuvant hormonal treatment may prove to be more effective than neoadjuvant chemotherapy.
- A complete response takes place when 100 percent of the cancer has responded to therapy. A partial response implies that 50 percent of the cancer has responded to therapy. However, the durability of the response is the critical attribute, except possibly in neoadjuvant therapy.
- Tamoxifen is known as an antiestrogen. It has three uses in breast cancer: (1) it has been used to effectively treat established breast cancer, (2) it can reduce the expected number of breast cancers in the contralateral breast, and (3) it can reduce the risk of getting breast cancer. It is the first "chemopreventive" agent that has been used in a clinical trial to prevent breast cancer.
- The STAR trial is testing the antiestrogen raloxifene to see if it is more effective than tamoxifen in preventing breast cancer.
- A relatively new class of drugs known as aromatase inhibitors may surpass tamoxifen in treating and (perhaps) preventing breast cancer.
- Aromatase inhibitors work by blocking the formation of estrogen, whereas drugs like tamoxifen interfere with the action of the previously formed estrogen.
- Biologic therapy has the advantage of treating only the specific cells to which it is directed. Thus, biologic therapeutic agents may not adversely affect normal cells and may have relatively few side effects. That makes them very attractive to both patients and oncology physicians.

Chapter 9 More Facts You Should Know

I am often asked, "What did I do to bring on this diagnosis of breast cancer? I live a good life—good home, good family, no smoking, no carousing, no unusual stress, so why me?"

The underlying questions really being asked are "What risk factors precipitated my diagnosis?" and "Can something be done about any one of those risk factors to reverse my diagnosis and maybe cure this cancer?"

Those are perfectly legitimate questions. So let's take a few moments to talk about risk factors and see if altering any one of them can prevent or cure breast cancer.

Risk Factors

What are risk factors? In the context of breast cancer, they are those elements in one's life that increase the probability of getting breast cancer. Risk factors fall into two groups: those you can't do anything about and those you can. As far as the first group is concerned, if you can't do anything, you can't. What about the second group, those risk factors that can be changed? Will it make a difference to try to modify any of them?

Here is a list of frequently found risk factors for breast cancer. (Note that age is not included in the list.)

- a personal history of breast cancer
- a family history of breast cancer
- a family history of breast cancer in male or female first-degree relatives
- atypical hyperplasia in your previous breast biopsy
- early menarche, late menopause
- no pregnancy
- exogenous estrogens
- exogenous estrogens plus progesterone (combined)
- obesity

The full list of breast cancer risk factors is very long. But bear in mind two facts to help you keep the subject of breast cancer risk in perspective: (1) The greatest risk for getting breast cancer is being over 60 years of age—and age isn't even on most lists; (2) *most women who have been diagnosed with breast cancer have no known risk factors.* Read that sentence twice. Armed with that information, let's look at major risk factors.

Age

Let's look at the risk factors you can't do anything about. Age is the single most important risk factor for breast cancer. Look at Figure 11 (in Chapter 7). It is a curve that shows the incidence of breast cancer versus age. The curve increases as age increases, reaching a peak at about 75–80 years of age. Note that essentially no cases of breast cancer are diagnosed between the ages of 20 and 24 years (although I recall a patient who was diagnosed to have breast cancer at age 18; her partner, a medical student, found the lump in her breast). A very substantial incidence of breast cancer occurs when a woman is older than 60 years. By the time a woman reaches that age, she is more likely than earlier in her life to be diagnosed with breast cancer. It is said by those who study breast cancer risk factors that when a woman reaches 60 years of age or older, she doesn't need to have any other risk factors; age is that important.

The decreased incidence of breast cancer in persons older than 75 years, shown in Figure 11, may result from the fact that this population is not screened regularly and consequently doesn't get diagnosed.

Can you do anything about your age? Not really. Short of suicide, you need to accept that age is a powerful risk factor for breast cancer, but one that you can't do anything about. What you *can* do is be vigilant about screening mammograms and breast exams as you get older.

Age does make a difference in the kind of treatment you are likely to get. It makes a difference whether you are premenopausal or postmenopausal—older or younger than approximately 50 years of age (see Chapter 8). It also makes a difference when you get routine mammograms (see Chapter 2).

Family History

Another risk factor you can't change is heredity. Once again, you can't do much about your genetic history. You *are* at a higher risk for breast cancer if you have more than one first-degree relative with breast cancer. Your mother, father (yes, men do get breast cancer), your brothers and sisters, grandparents (both sides of the family), aunts and even uncles (on both sides)—all are included in your family history.

If any of your parents, brothers and sisters, or grandparents were 35 years old or younger when they were diagnosed to have breast cancer, you may have either or both of the known breast cancer genes, BRCA 1 and BRCA 2. That is, you may have an inherited form of breast cancer.

Most breast cancers, the nonhereditary type, come from alterations or mutations in the nongermline body cells—cells that are not egg or sperm.

Alterations or mutations in the genetic material (DNA) of the egg or sperm can produce hereditary breast cancer, where the alterations remain in *all* cells of the offspring derived from that particular egg or sperm. Only a small number of persons—less than 5 percent of persons who have been diagnosed with breast cancer—have inherited breast cancer. It is usually diagnosed at a very young age, about 35 years. So a woman of 65 years, when she is diagnosed to have breast cancer, is *less likely* to harbor a breast cancer gene than a woman of 35 years with a family history of two first-degree relatives who were di-agnosed to have breast cancer at age 35 or younger.

Thus, it is not reasonable for someone to have genetic testing for breast cancer genes unless she or he fits a very specific category. Also, it is vital to recognize that even if you are found to have gene BRCA 1 or BRCA 2, it is not certain that you will develop breast cancer. The National Cancer Institute estimates that even if you carry gene BRCA 1 or BRCA 2, you have approximately an 80 percent, *not 100 percent*, chance of developing breast cancer by the time you reach 65 years of age. If you believe a glass is half full instead of half empty, you have approximately a 20 percent chance of *not* developing breast cancer by the time you are 65.

Testing for one of the breast cancer genes is expensive. Myriad Ge-netic Laboratories, a major laboratory that tests for BRCA 1 and 2, stated that as of February 1, 2001, it would cost $2,680 for a full BRCA 1 and 2 analysis. This is old information. By now, the cost may be even higher. Before you embark on a quest to determine whether you have a breast cancer gene, you should ask yourself two questions. Do you really want to spend the money to get this information? And once you get it, what will you do about it?

If you are confused and anxious about your risk of hereditary breast cancer, consult a genetic counselor (a breast geneticist) and discuss whether you should have genetic testing. He or she will examine your background and help you to understand your risk.

Estrogen

Unlike age and heredity, estrogen is a risk factor we can do something about. There are two kinds of estrogens about which we should be concerned. One is *exogenous* estrogen, which we take into our bodies. The other is *endogenous* estrogen—already within our bodies. For the purposes of this discussion, the distinction is unimportant; it is the *total* amount of the active form of estrogen in your body that is relevant.

No other environmental agent has been subjected to as much intense research as that which demonstrates that estrogens are implicated in causing breast cancer. Their role has been shown multiple times and in multiple ways. Scientists agree that estrogens are *promoters* of breast cancer. The direct cause of breast cancer, your genes, leads to a complex story that has still to be completely unraveled. For our purposes, we can say that estrogens can cause breast cancer—albeit weakly.

Anything that results in an increase of estrogen in your body appears to increase your risk of getting breast cancer. For example, obesity is regarded as a risk factor for breast cancer because the complex biochemistry of fat shows that fat can be converted to estrogen. Being obese appears to increase the total amount of estrogen in your body. Therefore, obesity appears to be a risk factor—an *indirect* risk factor—for breast cancer by virtue of its effect on estrogen, which is a *direct* risk factor.

Notice that many of the risk factors seem directly or indirectly related to estrogen. Many researchers claim that the risk is in the number of ovulations a woman undergoes. An increase in ovulations is associated with increased estrogen. The fewer ovulations a woman has before she becomes postmenopausal, the lower the probability that she will develop breast cancer. Conversely, the more ovulations she has, the greater the probability that she will develop breast cancer. For example, a woman's total number of ovulations decreases when she has a late menarche and early menopause. She doesn't ovulate during pregnancy. The reduced number of ovulations leads to a lower total amount of estrogen, which leads to a reduced risk of getting breast cancer.

Another critical fact is that estrogen has the capacity to promote the division of breast cancer cells both within the body and outside the body. In tissue culture, we can see this effect. It has significant implications for women who have been diagnosed with breast cancer, which is why we discontinue estrogen therapy in all women who have been so diagnosed regardless of the amount of estrogen being taken.

The antiestrogen tamoxifen has been used in the treatment of breast cancer for a long time. It works against both endogenous and exogenous estrogens. Antiestrogens, as the name suggests, are known to eliminate the action of estrogens. Researchers are now trying to determine whether we can manipulate the treatment of breast cancer so that estrogens can be totally eliminated. If so, could we then cure breast cancer? Could the elimination of estrogens prevent breast cancer?

Significantly reducing one risk factor such as estrogen has brought us a long way on the treatment track. It has even brought us a long way in our thinking about preventing breast cancer. Unfortunately, the cause of breast cancer is multifactorial. It takes more than one genetic mutation to cause breast cancer. More than one gene may be involved. Since estrogen is the product of a gene, and since more than one gene is involved in causing breast cancer, estrogen alone cannot be the single cause of breast cancer. That is one of the reasons why, in the first breast cancer prevention trial of the National Surgical Adjuvant trial for Breast Cancer Program (NSABP), the P_1 trial, tamoxifen reduced the incidence of breast cancer by approximately 50 percent, but not 100 percent.

Furthermore, approaches to treatment or prevention aimed at totally eliminating estrogen from the body are bound to stir controversy because of the positive roles estrogen plays outside the context of breast cancer. The years of increased breast cancer risk coincide with the years when women are losing estrogen. This coincidence poses a dilemma for women who want the significant benefits generated by estrogen.

Hormone Replacement Therapy and the Estrogen-Progesterone Story

I am asked frequently by postmenopausal women whether they should use any hormone replacement therapy (HRT), particularly in light of the Women's Health Initiative (WHI) study.

The acronym HRT refers to the use of hormones to replace those that decrease in number when a woman becomes postmenopausal. The term sometimes refers to the use of postmenopausal estrogen alone; it sometimes refers to the use of exogenous postmenopausal estrogen *plus* progesterone. When discussing HRT, you need to know which is being referred to.

The role of estrogen in hormone replacement therapy for postmenopausal women has been the subject of much debate. Several important studies have looked at issues such as the following: Is there a down side to taking exogenous estrogens? Do other drugs, when used with estrogen, act synergistically with the estrogen (creating a situation where the combined side effects, positive or negative, are greater than the additive side effects of the drugs separately?

Researchers are in agreement that the WHI study has shown that estrogen does not have the positive effect on the cardiovascular system that it was formerly thought to have. But it *does* have a positive effect on osteoporosis and also in eliminating symptoms of menopause such as hot flashes. Women with breast cancer who should not use estrogen but are worried about osteoporosis should know that other excellent drugs are available to them to protect against bone loss.

A great deal of media attention resulted when the WHI clinical trial *prematurely* closed the arm of the study in which both estrogen and progesterone were combined in a single pill known as Prempro (a combination of 0.625 milligram of premarin and 2.5 milligrams of progestin, a synthetic progesterone). Single pills are cheap and simple to use. Unfortunately, they contain fixed doses—as in the case of Prempro, where a fixed dose of premarin and a fixed dose of progesterone are used. The most commonly used dose of each was compounded into the pill. However, these might not be the optimal doses for you; for example, the premarin dose might be too high. You may be better served by a lower dose of premarin—for example, 0.3 mg.

The arm of the study in which Prempro was used was shut down at 5.2 years for several reasons, one being that the combination of estrogen with progesterone in Prempro was shown to cause a substantial increase of invasive breast cancer (Box 12). Progesterone proved to be the culprit. Actually, the increase in breast cancer was noted by the third year of the trial. After five years, it was felt that the risk was sufficient that maintaining the Prempro arm would do considerable harm.

The excessive number of breast cancer cases found was not a surprising result. Before the WHI trial began, and prior to the closing of the Prempro arm, an increasing number of medical papers in excellent peer-reviewed journals showed that the addition of progesterone to estrogen resulted in an increase in breast cancer. (These articles had

Box 12 Estrogen and Progesterone or Estrogen Alone?

Soon after the data on the Women's Health Initiative trial were released, the British published data from their Million Women Study which confirmed that the "combination of progestagen with oestrogen" in hormone replacement therapy (HRT) is associated with a "substantially greater risk of breast cancer than oestrogen-only therapy" (*The Lancet*, August 8, 2003).

Between 1996 and 2001, close to 1 million UK women aged 50–64 years were recruited into this British study. Half the women used the combination of estrogen *plus* progesterone. Totals of 9,364 breast cancers and 637 breast cancer deaths were registered. It is estimated that for every thousand postmenopausal women who took estrogen alone for ten years, five cases of estrogen-related breast cancer occurred. Compare this to nineteen cases of breast cancer associated with the combination of progesterone and estrogen. In other words, the combined estrogen and progesterone caused about four times as many breast cancers as estrogen alone.

In the United Kingdom, the use of HRT (estrogen alone or the combination of estrogen and progesterone) over ten years has resulted in an estimated twenty thousand breast cancers, of which fifteen thousand are believed to be associated with the combination of estrogen plus progesterone.

impressed me enough that for many years I had been advising women not to use the combination of estrogen and progesterone.)

As long as some procedure is controversial, don't do it. Don't assume your doctor is better informed about new drugs than you are. Drug companies sell agents with names other than progesterone and recommend that they be taken to avoid cancer of the uterus. Many physicians, for example, have been told that micronized progesterone will not lead to breast cancer when taken with estrogen. Micronized progesterone, however, is still progesterone. Read the fine print on any package insert to be sure you are not ingesting progesterone under a different, attractive name. Don't be fooled into taking progesterone *in any form* along with estrogen.

I repeat: estrogen has been shown to stimulate the division of breast cancer cells, both within and outside the body. *So does progesterone.*

Estrogen can cause breast cancer, although it is a weak carcinogen for that disease. It also has been shown to cause cancer of the uterus (endometrial cancer)—again, as a weak carcinogen. The endometrial cancer caused by estrogen generally is found early in a low stage and its *grade* is usually very low. This low-grade, low-stage cancer is potentially cured by a hysterectomy.

The fact that progesterone protects the uterus from the cancer-inducing effect of estrogen has been known for many years. What is not so well known is that *the addition of progesterone to estrogen can cause a significant increase in breast cancer.* The cancer of the uterus that results from estrogen use is, like endometrial cancer, low stage, low grade, and potentially curable by hysterectomy. Breast cancer, on the other hand, is likely to be lethal. What kind of trade-off is that? Nonetheless, many physicians still prescribe a combination of estrogen and progesterone for postmenopausal women who have not had a hysterectomy (their uterus is intact).

Prior to the closing of the Prempro arm of the WHI study, sales of the pill were strong. Subsequent sales have been greatly reduced. The heavy media attention to the discontinuance of Prempro in the WHI trial left many women confused. Should they continue Prempro? Should they use estrogen alone? Should they not use hormones at all? Their physicians were confused, too.

What many fail to realize is that the study involving the use of estrogen alone has *not* been closed. The WHI trial retained the arm in which estrogen alone is used for HRT in women who have *already undergone a hysterectomy*. The WHI study thus far has demonstrated no significant untoward effects of estrogen alone, and it has confirmed that estrogen is a weak carcinogen for breast cancer. Estrogen alone in women who have had hysterectomies is still regarded as appropriate hormone replacement, so long as it is not used to overcome the negative effects of cardiovascular disease.

It is worth mentioning again that estrogen can eliminate hot flashes in the postmenopausal woman. Hot flashes can be uncomfortable; in fact, they can be debilitating. They can interfere with sleep, rendering the victim exhausted. They have a similar effect on the woman's partner. Because the victim of hot flashes spends the night pulling the bedcovers on and off, her partner also becomes sleep deprived and exhausted. Estrogen can eliminate this problem and improve sleep for both individuals.

Here is my advice to menopausal and postmenopausal women: *If you have never had a diagnosis of breast cancer* and wish to take estrogens for HRT, use the lowest possible dose to eliminate symptoms such as hot flashes. Don't use estrogen for a prolonged period. If you must take estrogen, have a yearly vaginal ultrasound (to look at the lining of the uterus—the endometrium—where cancer of the uterus develops). If the ultrasound shows a thickened endometrium, I recommend an endometrial biopsy to help you determine whether you have cancer of the uterus.

If you have been diagnosed to have breast cancer, *throw your estrogens away* and never use them again, regardless of the form of estrogen —pill, skin cream, etc.—you are using. Estrogens are known to stimulate the division of breast cancer cells both within and outside the body. Even if many years have passed since your breast cancer was diagnosed, even if your breast cancer was noninvasive or in the very early phase of stage I, even if the estrogen you take is a very low dose, why take the chance of developing metastatic breast cancer?

Many women who have had *pre*menopausal breast cancer, when they become *post*menopausal, have unremitting and severe hot flashes. They have been told correctly that they cannot take estrogen because estrogen promotes cell division. These women become desperate for relief, and they know estrogen can relieve these symptoms. I sympathize with these women. I know from personal experience, even though I did not have a diagnosis of breast cancer, that severe hot flashes are extremely uncomfortable and can interfere with quality of life. My advice to these afflicted women is to be strong and to recognize that hot flashes won't last forever, but that metastatic breast cancer can significantly shorten your "forever."

If you have had breast cancer, be cautious. Know that estrogens come in many forms. *Read the labels.* Estrogens can be found in face creams that are not manufactured in the United States and are advertised as giving your skin a youthful appearance. Estrogens are well absorbed from the skin into your body. Thus, estrogen-containing creams can lead to systemic estrogen, totally undesirable for the woman who has had breast cancer.

Many women with breast cancer become extremely unhappy when told to throw away their estrogens. They believe they look and feel young because of their estrogen, but estrogen has *not* been shown to be the secret of eternal youth, or to be responsible for youthful skin.

Even innocuous-sounding soy products contain high concentrations of plant-produced estrogens called phytoestrogens. As Shakespeare wrote, "a rose by any other name" . . . Phytoestrogens are still estrogens and still have estrogenic effects. Therefore, take soy products with care and do not consume excessive amounts of soy preparations. Unfortunately, health food products such as soy are unregulated, and you may have no knowledge of what or how much estrogen from soy you are taking. Anything bought in a health food store that claims to eliminate hot flashes gives you a clue that it contains estrogen-like substances.

Men and Breast Cancer

Yes, men can get breast cancer. Each year about 1,200 men are diagnosed to have breast cancer. This figure amounts to less than 1 percent of diagnosed breast cancer.

Male and female breast cancers are essentially similar. As in women, most male breast cancers are diagnosed when men are between 60 and 70 years of age, although breast cancer can occur in men at any age. The types of breast cancer, the treatments, and the survival rates are all the same.

However, the *diagnosis* of male breast cancer is somewhat different. Because male breast cancer is so rare, screening mammography is not done. If an abnormality is felt in the male breast, diagnostic tests (including mammography) should be carried out, with pathology providing the final, definitive diagnosis.

The treatment and aftercare of male breast cancer are essentially the same as for women. Thus, anything that I have said in this book regarding women applies also to men.

Remember . . .

- Age is the single most important risk factor for breast cancer.
- Risk factors for breast cancer fall into two groups: those you can do

something about (such as estrogens) and those you can't (such as age and heredity).

- You can do something about the total amount of estrogen in your body.
- Estrogen is one of the causes of breast cancer—albeit a weak cause.
- Both estrogen and progesterone can cause breast cancer cells to divide.
- The combination of estrogen and progesterone creates a huge risk factor for breast cancer. The arm of the WHI study that utilized the combination pill Prempro was prematurely closed, in part because of the large number of breast cancers that occurred. The responsible agent was progesterone.
- The British Million Women Study confirmed that the combination of estrogen and progesterone caused a huge incidence of breast cancer.
- My advice to postmenopausal women who do not have breast cancer is to take estrogen at the lowest possible dose to eliminate symptoms of menopause (like hot flashes), and for the shortest time possible. My advice to those women who have had breast cancer, no matter how long ago, is not to take estrogen in any form.
- Less than 1 percent of diagnosed breast cancers are in men. Treatment and aftercare for male breast cancer are the same as for women.

Chapter 10 Transition Time

As the years pass, what happens to those of us who have been treated for breast cancer? Long after we become "survivors," do we go about our daily activities as usual or are we forever scarred? What happened to our significant others during this battle? Were they too scarred by this experience? What about other loved ones—parents, siblings, friends? And children—what about them? If they were living in the same house, how could they escape? Didn't they hear the vomiting? Didn't they see the bald head? Didn't they experience the anxiety of waiting for the biopsy results? Could they really turn off our suffering? Can we ever turn it off?

A great deal is known about our emotions and behavior during diagnosis and active treatment for breast cancer. Less is known about our emotions and behavior at the time treatment ends, although some research on that period has reached the scientific literature. We know a great deal about the subsequent time, the survivor period, although much of our knowledge is anecdotal. It is the *transition* period—when

Decision Tree 8 Return Visits after Treatment Is Finished

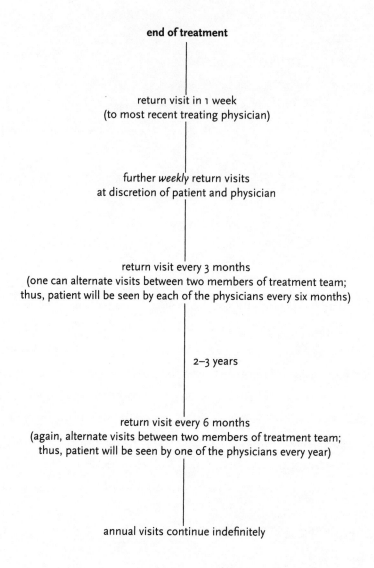

end of treatment

return visit in 1 week
(to most recent treating physician)

further *weekly* return visits
at discretion of patient and physician

return visit every 3 months
(one can alternate visits between two members of treatment team;
thus, patient will be seen by each of the physicians every six months)

2–3 years

return visit every 6 months
(again, alternate visits between two members of treatment team;
thus, patient will be seen by one of the physicians every year)

annual visits continue indefinitely

we move from being a patient to becoming independent—about which we know the least.

Each of these three periods—(1) the diagnostic and treatment period, (2) the transition period, and (3) the survivor period—involves its own emotional and physical challenges. Period 1 has a well-defined beginning and end. Period 2 has a well-defined beginning but a poorly defined end. Period 3 occurs long after treatment ends and lasts five or more years.

When the psychosocial and physical aspects of the three periods are examined, the results differ. Yet in each of four groups of patients (lumpectomy with or without chemotherapy, and mastectomy with or without chemotherapy; radiation and hormonal treatment given in each group), the *emotional* functioning of all the patients was the same at the end of each period. Contrary to expectation, regardless of how rigorous and complex their treatment had been, women ended up emotionally the same by the time treatment ended. What stood out was that women who had had chemotherapy as part of their treatment regimen, regardless of their surgical treatment, complained of more physical symptoms than women who had not had chemotherapy. Among the complaints were generalized aches and pains, vaginal dryness and painful intercourse, muscle stiffness, and decreased arm mobility. These physical symptoms, for some investigators, had prognostic significance.

In this chapter, I focus on the period that is least understood—the transition period. It begins with the end of treatment and generally lasts up to about twelve months. It truly is a time of transition, a time of change, a time when one moves from being a patient to becoming independent. It can be very stressful.

In general, patients are seen more frequently soon after treatment is over, with return visits being spaced at increasingly longer intervals as the patient enters the survivor period (after one year). I suggest that you be seen one week after treatment is over and then every three months during the transition period (alternating between two physician members of your treatment team is acceptable if these two physicians are in close contact). Two to three years after treatment has ended, the return visits can be spaced at six-month intervals, again alternating between two members of your treatment team as an option. When you are well into the survivor period, you can be seen once a year. This yearly return visit should be routine for the rest of your life (Decision Tree 8). Of course, this program can be modified to suit your individual needs and the requirements of your treating physicians.

At the end of treatment, many patients feel as if a safety net has been withdrawn. They are going from a time of seeing their oncologists and staff very frequently to a time of seeing them infrequently. In my practice as a radiation oncologist, I became accustomed to seeing patients who had completed their daily radiation treatments return after a few days with some sort of excuse, just to see us again.

Many women worry that a recurrence of their tumor is more likely now that active treatment has ended. This worry can be overwhelming and can markedly interfere with the patient's quality of life. Still others are disappointed that they don't feel totally well when treatment is over, certainly not as well as they felt before they were diagnosed with breast cancer.

More important, close family members who had altered their own lives are disappointed because they expect the former patient to resume the tasks and responsibilities they performed prior to breast cancer treatment.

Women who, *with a tremendous effort,* coped well during treatment may feel extremely disappointed that they cannot carry out their pretreatment tasks and responsibilities. As a result, they may feel depressed and even more anxious than before. Many have double emotions: relief that treatment is over, but extreme anxiety about the future.

Some women have problems with their self-image and the image others have of them—in particular, they worry about the reaction of their children to their diagnosis of breast cancer.

Physicians and their staff are generally very helpful in describing the acute side effects of treatment. But few know or take the time to acknowledge to the patient that sometimes the side effects of treatment last well into the transition period. If you, the patient, don't know about these lingering effects, you may worry that the symptoms are harbingers of a recurrence. You may not know which symptoms you should monitor and report to the physician who next sees you. In fact, you may be confused about which physician you should see and when. This uncertainty can renew the feeling of loss of control.

Even without supporting data, many experienced physicians caution their patients that *recovery* from the acute effects of treatment will take about as long as the treatment itself. This estimate is probably correct.

With the end of active treatment you may need your family members and friends more than ever. It should be obvious to loved ones that they need to give as much emotional support as possible, rather than withdraw support because you are becoming independent. *Family members and friends should be aware that you need their support even more now.* If they aren't, they should be made aware. The need for family and friends may be greatest after active treatment is over.

All the persons close to a breast cancer survivor have an important role in maintaining the quality of life of the survivor. Get as much support as you can, wherever you find it.

It helps everyone to know what to expect. You may or may not experience all of the side effects and aftereffects of treatment, but being prepared can make a difference in *how* you experience them. Monitor your symptoms if you have any, and ask your physician to consider prescribing for them if they are particularly troublesome.

Many in the transition period are plagued by fatigue. We certainly don't know what causes fatigue, but it is undeniable that many women are severely fatigued by the end of treatment. Since their exhaustion lasts well into the transition period, patients are concerned and wonder if it will ever go away. And of course, many worry that fatigue presages persistent or recurrent disease.

Other common effects include alopecia (hair loss), abnormal menses, and generalized aches and pains. If any of these side effects (including fatigue) are prolonged, don't hesitate to tell your physician about them.

Sexual functioning, glossed over in the recent past, may still receive too little attention. It is a significant aspect of quality of life that should be discussed with your physician. If you have problems with sexual function *after* treatment, and discussions with your physician are not adequate for you and your partner, you may wish to see a sex counselor. The diagnosis and treatment for breast cancer take their toll on both partners.

In a recent large survey, approximately 60 percent of women reported that they were sexually active by the end of treatment. When asked to describe the serious to moderate limitations on their sexual activity, about 7 percent reported that their *partners* were "too tired" and another 7 percent reported that their *partners* were not interested. Was patient fatigue somehow implicated? In this same survey, approximately half of the women who received chemotherapy for breast cancer, regardless of the type of surgery, reported more negative effects on their sex life than the group of women who did not have chemotherapy. Of those women who reported poor sexual functioning, inadequate vaginal lubrication and the resulting painful intercourse accounted for a significant amount of sexual dysfunction. Unfortunately, these problems persist and worsen with time and age.

With any symptom, ask your physician if it is a treatment-related problem or if it might have another, possibly treatable, cause. One frequent complaint, for example, is "difficulty concentrating." This can be a treatment-related problem or it can reflect a depression. After evaluating the problem, your physician might consider referring you to a psychiatrist. That physician in turn might elicit the answer and possibly prescribe appropriate medication.

Problems related to your self-image and the image that others have of you (or are expected to have of you) should not be ignored. Your children's reaction to you, the affection and sexual interest your partner shows you during the transition period, can profoundly affect your quality of life. Is your partner as overtly loving as before your diagnosis and treatment? Are your children, especially your daughters, acting differently? Mothers diagnosed to have breast cancer often complain to me that their teenaged daughters have become uncooperative and unloving. This is not surprising; many daughters are angry with their mothers for "giving them breast cancer" and all that goes with it.

Partners, too, undergo severe changes to their quality of life after their significant other undergoes the physical and emotional trauma of having and being treated for breast cancer. Your partner may outwardly seem to be relatively unaffected, but together you *both* have gone through a damaging period. Whether the result is a closer bonding or a less close relationship, your partner is changed forever too.

Your personal attitudes, such as fighting spirit and sense of humor, can be key. They may make more of a difference than we physicians know. So, do keep a positive attitude—and fight!

What about support groups? Clearly, they perform a vital function. But not everyone is emotionally capable of making effective use of support groups. Look at a potential support group carefully. Ask yourself, "How will I react if a member of this group dies?" Or, "Is this really a positive experience for me? How will I feel if I see a person worse off than I am? Will I identify with another member of the group who had a similar stage of breast cancer at the time of diagnosis? What if that person has symptoms that I don't have as yet?" Only you can determine whether a particular support group will be helpful to you. *If you think it will not be, don't go.*

As you progress through the transition period to survivorship, think even more about what you can do to protect yourself from a recurrence. Until now, you may have felt powerless. All kinds of people have been telling you what to do: your doctors, nurses, social workers, even schedulers. Now it's time to tell yourself what to do.

For starters, you can tell yourself to eat better. At no time in your life is your nutrition as important as it is now, when you have completed active treatment and are heading into a relatively normal life. If your diet was 2,300 calories or more per day, reduce that number to 1,800 or fewer. Your new diet should be low in saturated fats and high in such cruciferous (smelly) vegetables as broccoli, cauliflower, and cabbage. Recognize that a low normal weight is helpful to your other body systems. Think of what it may mean for breast cancer. A low normal weight means less body fat and a reduction in total body estrogen—which may go a long way toward combating a recurrence.

You also can exercise. Preliminary data suggest that thirty minutes of moderate exercise five days a week should reduce the breast cancer recurrence rate in postmenopausal women.

What else can you actively do for yourself? Reread Chapter 9 on the risks and prevention of breast cancer. In particular, note the short list of risk factors. Even though not much is known about most of these factors as the cause of breast cancer, this shouldn't dissuade you from changing your environment or lifestyle to combat a potential recurrence.

Your emotional state is extremely important. I can't tell you that emotional serenity will reduce a recurrence rate. But I can say unequivocally that it is energizing to wake up each day and feel that life is precious. I can also say that a positive frame of mind is healthy.

You have gone through so much during your screening, diagnosis, decision making about treatment, and finally treatment itself. If you follow the course of the average person who has been treated for breast cancer, you have emerged from this trauma emotionally intact. Now that you have moved through the transition period and are a survivor, you realize that you are now better equipped emotionally to handle the rest of your life.

I congratulate you! I wish you well. Always remember, you are not a statistic.

Resources

Breast Cancer Resources

American Breast Cancer Foundation, www.abcf.org; 1055 Taylor Avenue, Suite 201A, Baltimore, MD 21286; phone (410) 825-9388; toll free (877) 539-2543; fax (410) 825-4395; email bcancertw@aol.com. The ABCF mission is to provide early-detection education and screening services to those in need, regardless of age, race, sex, or financial challenge. The foundation promotes health education and provides life-saving breast cancer screening assistance through outreach events such as the Remote Area Medical (RAM) Expeditions held in impoverished communities in rural areas of the United States.

Breast Cancer Fund, www.breastcancerfund.org; 2107 O'Farrell Street, San Francisco, CA 94115; phone (415) 346-8223; fax (415) 346-2975; email info@breastcancerfund.org. Identifies the environmental links to breast cancer through reports, fact sheets, and other research materials; educates the public on how to reduce exposure to cancer-causing chemicals. Website helpful to learn about prevention, advocacy, and athletic fundraisers.

www.cdc.gov/cancer/nbccedp/contacts.htm. This Centers for Disease Control website lists where in each state free or low-cost mammograms are available.

FDA Certified Mammography Facilities, www.accessdata.fda.gov/scripts/cdrh/cfdocs/cfMQSA/mqsa.cfm. This website will search for certified mammography facilities in your area.

Imaginis, www.imaginis.com; Imaginis Corporation, Attn: J. Molloy, PO Box 27018, Greenville, SC 29616; email learnmore@imaginis.com. An award-winning resource for news and information on breast cancer prevention, screening, diagnosis and treatment, and related women's health topics. The home page lists breast health topics, and the content is created by an independent team of breast health specialists to ensure that it is up to date and accurate. Complicated medical terms are explained in everyday language to help readers understand their options.

LifeLines, www.shanti.org; 730 Polk Street, Third Floor, San Francisco, CA 94109; phone (415) 674-4780; email lifelines@shanti.org. A project of the Breast Cancer Fund and Shanti, LifeLines provides culturally sensitive services for low-income women affected by breast cancer. The services include peer support, food delivery, help with chores, transportation, and free activities.

National Breast and Cervical Cancer Early Detection Program, www.cdc.gov/cancer/nbccedp/index.htm. This Centers for Disease Control website is directed at low-income women, providing them with information about early-detection mammography rescreening.

National Alliance of Breast Cancer Organizations (NABCO), www.nabco.org. NABCO was a network of approximately four hundred organizations, the leading nonprofit breast cancer information and education resource in the United States, and a national force in patient advocacy. NABCO permanently discontinued operations on June 30, 2004, concluding eighteen years of pioneering programs, leadership, and service to the breast cancer community. The American Society of Clinical Oncology (www.asco.org) now hosts NABCO's website, where NABCO will post updates and other communications.

National Breast Cancer Coalition, 1101 17th Street, NW, Suite 1300, Washington, DC 20036; phone (800) 622-2838. A grassroots advocacy group that publishes a "Guide to Quality Breast Cancer Care."

Rose Kushner Breast Cancer Advisory Center, www.rkbcac.org; PO Box 757, Malaga Cove, CA 90274. Website provides an extensive array of information about breast cancer. Rose Kushner, one of the founders of the now-disbanded National Alliance of Breast Cancer Organizations, created this site.

Susan G. Komen Breast Cancer Foundation, www.komen.org. Website includes an excellent breast self-exam video and a locational directory of Komen affiliates. Komen affiliates focus on the Race for the Cure, although the website provides extensive information about breast cancer.

Women's Information Network (WIN) Against Breast Cancer, www.winabc.org; 536 S. Second Avenue, Suite K, Covina, CA 91723-3043; phone (866) 2WINABC. This site contains cancer resources and information for newly diagnosed patients.

Yale–New Haven Breast Center, www.yalenewhavenbreastcenter.org; 800 Howard Avenue, Lower Level, PO Box 208062, New Haven, CT 06520-8062; phone (203) 785-2328; fax (203) 785-2329; email breast.center@yale.edu. A combined resource of the Yale Medical Group, The Physicians of Yale University, Yale–New Haven Hospital, and Yale Cancer Center.

Y-Me, www.y-me.org, National Organization for Breast Cancer. This website is comprehensive and easy to use. Information is offered in Vietnamese, Korean, Chinese, and Spanish. The 24-hour hotline is (800) 221-2141 or (800) 986-9505 (Spanish) and interpreters provide information in more than 140 languages. The hotline can match you with someone who has survived breast cancer and has a similar cancer history. The site also offers a free monthly one-hour teleconference featuring a health care professional who presents a topic concerning breast cancer, followed by a question and answer session.

www.ywca.org. Through EncorePlus, many YWCAs connect women to free or low-cost mammograms. This main website has links to YWCAs around the country and internationally.

Additional Useful Websites

www.breastcancer.net. Gives useful links to breast cancer sources and provides information for Spanish speakers.

www.breastcancer.org; 111 Forrest Avenue 1R, Narberth, PA 19072. A non-profit organization for breast cancer education. Website includes recordings of celebrities defining medical terms related to breast cancer.

www.drkoop.com; women's section at www.drkoop.com/template. asp?page=channel&ap=93&cid=1953 provides breast cancer updates and answers.

www.oncolink.org. This cancer link provides a page entitled Ask the Expert, on which you can post questions to breast cancer experts.

General Cancer Resources

American Cancer Society; phone (800) 227-2345. Spanish-speaker option available; around-the-clock availability. Offers special programs for people with breast cancer and a cancer survivors' network.

American Society of Clinical Oncology (ASCO), www.asco.org. A professional organization representing physicians who treat people with cancer. See also National Alliance of Breast Cancer Organizations (NABCO), in the Breast Cancer Resources section of this list.

Avon Breast Cancer Crusade, www.avoncrusade.com. Raises both funds and awareness regarding access to care and finding a cure for breast cancer.

Cancer Care, Inc., www.cancercare.org; phone (800) 813-HOPE (4637). Offices in New York, New Jersey, and Connecticut. Website provides cancer care services such as links to online, telephone, and on-site support groups and can help you locate such resources as drug assistance programs in your state. Offers free counseling and telephone educational workshops.

Cancer Chat, www.oncochat.org. A global support network for cancer patients and their families. Does not offer medical advice or counseling.

www.cancereducation.com. Website allows you to search for clinical trials near you and physicians who are listed according to cancer specialty.

National Cancer Institute, www.nci.nih.gov; phone (800) 4-CANCER. Website can be translated into Spanish; provides information on treatment, prevention, genetics, causes, screening and testing, clinical trials, breast cancer literature, statistics, research, and related information.

National Cancer Institute's Cancer Information Service, http://cis.nci.nih.gov. A free national information and education network provided by the United States National Cancer Institute.

National Institutes of Health, www.nih.gov; 9000 Rockville Pike, Bethesda, MD 20892; main telephone number (301) 496-4000; toll-free cancer numbers (800) 422-6237, (800)-332-8615 (TTY). Website provides A–Z list of cancer topics. Breast cancer link includes news on research advances, a cancer dictionary, facts about breast cancer, and several links to information in Spanish.

Women's Cancer Network, www.wcn.org. Designed to keep women informed about gynecologic cancer and to assist women who have developed cancer.

Breast Cancer–Related Resources

American College of Radiology, www.acr.org; 1891 Preston White Drive, Weston, VA 20191-4397; general e-mail info@acr.org. Website provides a list of accredited facilities for mammography in your area.

American Society of Plastic Surgeons, www.plasticsurgery.org. Lists board-certified plastic surgeons in your area and provides basic information about breast reconstructive surgery. Includes online referral service.

ICI Pharmaceutical Nolvadex Patient Assistance Program. Helps financially eligible women receive tamoxifen.

Myriad Genetics, Inc. Provides testing for BRCA-1 and BRCA-2.

National Lymphedema Network, Inc. Information on how to choose a lymphedema specialist.

Onotech. Testing of cancer cells for drug resistance and sensitivity.

Rational Therapeutics Cancer Laboratories, www.rationaltherapeutics. com. Provides cancer therapies tailored to the individual patient by determining, in the laboratory, which drugs are most effective for cell death.

Single Point of Contact, www.biooncology.com/bioonc/pr_ri.jsp. Provides a flexible reimbursement service to underinsured or uninsured patients using Genentech BioOncology products in their treatment.

Resources Developed for Minorities

Lesbian Community Cancer Project, www.lccp.org; 4753 N. Broadway, Suite 602, Chicago, IL 60640; phone (773) 561-4662; fax (773) 561-1830; email info@lccp.org. An advocacy group that aims to ensure that lesbian, bisexual, and transgender women have appropriate and accessible health care in a supportive and bias-free environment.

Mary-Helen Mautner Project for Lesbians with Cancer, www.
mautnerproject.org/index.html. Promotes lesbian health through research, advocacy, direct support, and education.

National Black Leadership Initiative on Cancer, www.nblic.org. A project
of the National Cancer Institute established to create cancer control, prevention, and research and training programs for minority and under-
served populations.

Sisters Network, Inc., www.sistersnetworkinc.org. A national African
American breast cancer survivorship program that gives statistics on
African American women and breast cancer, and locates Sisters Network
affiliates around the country.

Specific Peer-Reviewed Medical Information for Professionals

American Association for Cancer Research, www.aacr.org; 615 Chestnut
Street, 17th Floor, Philadelphia, PA 19106-4404; phone (215) 440-9300;
fax (215) 440-9313. A society of more than 22,000 laboratory and clinical
scientists engaged in all areas of cancer research in the United States and
more than sixty other countries. Publishes five major peer-reviewed scientific journals: *Cancer Research; Clinical Cancer Research; Molecular Cancer Therapeutics; Molecular Cancer Research;* and *Cancer Epidemiology, Bio-
markers, and Prevention.*

Breast Cancer Online, www.bco.org. The stated purpose of this site is "to
facilitate timely access to new trends and topical information in breast
cancer for healthcare professionals." The typical user of this site works in
the field of breast cancer research and treatment, so it is geared toward
health-care professionals. Patients seeking guidance can refer to the section called "Patient Information."

Medical Books

V. DeVita Jr., S. Hellman, and S. Rosenberg, Eds., *Cancer: Principles and Practices of Oncology,* 6th edition. Philadelphia: Lippincott-Raven, 2001.

J. Harris et al., Eds., *Diseases of the Breast,* 3rd edition. Philadelphia: Lippincott Williams & Wilkins, 2004.

M. Lippman, A. Lichter, and D. Dansforth, Eds., *Diagnosis and Management of Breast Cancer.* Philadelphia: Saunders, 1988.

P. Rosen and H. Oberman, *Tumors of the Mammary Gland.* Washington, DC: Armed Forces Institute of Pathology, 1993.

Medical Journals

Cancer Research. Publishes original research in cancer and cancer-related biomedical studies, including cell and tumor biology, experimental therapeutics, immunology, molecular biology, and prevention.

Clinical Cancer Research. Publishes original research on prevention, characterization, diagnosis, and treatment of human cancer.

Journal of Clinical Oncology. Publishes original research and reviews concerning supportive care and quality of life, cancer prevention, and clinical pharmacology.

The Journal of the National Cancer Institute. Publishes original cancer research from around the world. *The Journal of the National Cancer Institute* is not affiliated with the United States National Cancer Institute.

The Lancet. Publishes original research and reviews in all aspects of human health, with an international focus.

The New England Journal of Medicine. Publishes on a wide variety of topics, with an emphasis on internal medicine.

The Oncologist. Publishes original research, reviews, and commentaries addressing diagnosis, treatment, and quality of life of the cancer patient.

Proceedings of the National Academy of Sciences. Publishes the research reports, commentaries, perspectives, reviews, papers, and actions of the United States National Academy of Sciences.

Science. This weekly magazine, published by the American Association for the Advancement of Science, offers original research, reviews, and analyses of current research and science policy in all areas of science (not just health).

Seminars in Oncology. Publishes current reviews of developments in diagnosis and management of cancer patients.

National Cancer Institute–Designated Cancer Centers, by State

Alabama
UAB Comprehensive Cancer Center
University of Alabama, Birmingham
1824 Sixth Avenue South, Room 237
Birmingham, AL 35293-3300
Phone (205) 934-5077; fax (205) 975-7428
(Comprehensive Cancer Center)

Arizona
Arizona Cancer Center
University of Arizona
1501 North Campbell Avenue
Tucson, AZ 85724
Phone (520) 626-7925; fax (520) 626-2284
(Comprehensive Cancer Center)

California
City of Hope National Medical Center and
Beckman Research Institute
1500 East Duarte Road

Duarte, CA 91010-3000

Phone (626) 359-8111, X 64297; fax (626) 930-5394

(Comprehensive Cancer Center)

Cancer Center

<u>Salk Institute</u>

10010 North Torrey Pines Road

La Jolla, CA 92037

Phone (858) 453-4100, X 1386; fax (858) 457-4765

(Cancer Center)

Cancer Research Center

<u>The Burnham Institute</u>

10901 North Torrey Pines Road

La Jolla, CA 92037

Phone (858) 646-3100; fax (858) 713-6274

(Cancer Center)

<u>Rebecca and John Moores UCSD Cancer Center</u>

University of California, San Diego

9500 Gilman Drive

La Jolla, CA 92093-0658

Phone (858) 822-1222; fax (858) 822-1207

(Comprehensive Cancer Center)

<u>Jonsson Comprehensive Cancer Center</u>

University of California, Los Angeles

Factor Building, Room 8-684

10833 Le Conte Avenue

Los Angeles, CA 90095-1781

Phone (310) 825-5268; fax (310) 206-5553

(Comprehensive Cancer Center)

Norris Comprehensive Cancer Center
University of Southern California
1441 Eastlake Avenue, NOR 8302L
Los Angeles, California 90089-9181
Phone (323) 865-0816; fax (323) 865-0102
(Comprehensive Cancer Center)

Chao Family Comprehensive Cancer Center
University of California, Irvine
101 The City Drive
Building 23, Route 81, Room 406
Orange, CA 92868
Phone (714) 456-6310; fax (714) 456-2240
(Comprehensive Cancer Center)

UC Davis Cancer Center
University of California, Davis
4501 X Street, Suite 3003
Sacramento, CA 95817
Phone (916) 734-5800; fax (916) 451-4464
(Clinical Cancer Center)

UCSF Comprehensive Cancer Center and Cancer Research Institute
University of California, San Francisco
2340 Sutter Street, Box 0128
San Francisco, CA 94115-0128
Phone (415) 502-1710; fax (415) 502-1712
(Comprehensive Cancer Center)

Colorado
University of Colorado Cancer Center
University of Colorado Health Science Center
4200 East 9th Avenue, Box B188

Denver, CO 80262

Phone (303) 315-3007; fax (303) 315-3304

(Comprehensive Cancer Center)

Connecticut

Yale Cancer Center

Yale University School of Medicine

333 Cedar Street, Box 208028

New Haven, CT 06520-8028

Phone (203) 785-4371; fax (203) 785-4116

(Comprehensive Cancer Center)

District of Columbia

Lombardi Cancer Research Center

Georgetown University Medical Center

3800 Reservoir Road, NW

Washington, DC 20007

Phone (202) 687-2110; fax (202) 687-6402

(Comprehensive Cancer Center)

Florida

H. Lee Moffitt Cancer Center and Research Institute

University of South Florida

12902 Magnolia Drive, MCC-CEO

Tampa, FL 33612-9497

Phone (813) 615-4261; fax (813) 615-4258

(Comprehensive Cancer Center)

Hawaii

Cancer Research Center of Hawaii

University of Hawaii, Manoa

1236 Lauhala Street

Honolulu, HI 96813

Phone (808) 586-3013; fax (808) 586-3052

(Clinical Cancer Center)

Illinois

University of Chicago Cancer Research Center

5841 South Maryland Avenue, MC 2115

Chicago, IL 60637-1470

Phone (773) 702-9306; fax (773) 702-3002

(Clinical Cancer Center)

Robert H. Lurie Comprehensive Cancer Center

Northwestern University

303 East Chicago Avenue

Olson Pavilion 8250

Chicago, IL 60611

Phone (312) 908-5250; fax (312) 908-1372

(Comprehensive Cancer Center)

Indiana

Indiana University Cancer Center

Indiana Cancer Pavilion

535 Barnhill Drive, Room 455

Indianapolis, IN 46202-5289

Phone (317) 278-0070; fax (317) 278-0074

(Clinical Cancer Center)

Purdue University Cancer Center

Hansen Life Sciences Research Building

South University Street

West Lafayette, IN 47907-1524

Phone (765) 494-9129; fax (765) 494-9193

(Cancer Center)

Iowa

Holden Comprehensive Cancer Center

University of Iowa

5970 "Z" JPP

200 Hawkins Drive

Iowa City, IA 52242

Phone (319) 353-8620; fax (319) 353-8988

(Comprehensive Cancer Center)

Maine

Jackson Laboratory

600 Main Street

Bar Harbor, ME 04609-0800

Phone (207) 288-6041; fax (207) 288-6044

(Cancer Center)

Maryland

Sidney Kimmel Comprehensive Cancer Center

Johns Hopkins University

401 North Broadway

Weinberg Building, Suite 1100

Baltimore, MD 21231

Phone (410) 955-8822; fax (410) 955-6787

(Comprehensive Cancer Center)

Massachusetts

Dana-Farber/Harvard Cancer Center

Dana-Farber Cancer Institute

44 Binney Street, Room 1628

Boston, MA 02115

Phone (617) 632-4266; fax (617) 632-2161

(Comprehensive Cancer Center)

Center for Cancer Research
Massachusetts Institute of Technology
77 Massachusetts Avenue, Room E17-110
Cambridge, MA 02139-4307
Phone (617) 253-8511; fax (617) 253-0262
(Cancer Center)

Michigan
Comprehensive Cancer Center
University of Michigan
6302 CGC/0942
1500 East Medical Center Drive
Ann Arbor, MI 48109-0942
Phone (734) 936-1831; fax (734) 615-3947
(Comprehensive Cancer Center)

Meyer L. Prentis Comprehensive Cancer Center of Metropolitan Detroit
Barbara Ann Karmanos Cancer Institute
Wayne State University
4100 John R
Detroit, MI 48201
Phone (313) 993-7770; fax (313) 993-7165
(Comprehensive Cancer Center)

Minnesota
University of Minnesota Cancer Center
MMC 806, 420 Delaware Street, SE
Minneapolis, MN 55455
Phone (612) 624-8484; fax (612) 626-3069
(Comprehensive Cancer Center)

Mayo Clinic College of Medicine
Mayo Clinic Rochester

200 First Street, SW

Rochester, MN 55905

Phone (507) 284-3753; fax (507) 284-9349

(Comprehensive Cancer Center)

Missouri

Siteman Cancer Center

Washington University School of Medicine

660 South Euclid Avenue, Campus Box 8109

St. Louis, MO 63110

Phone (314) 362-8020; fax (314) 454-1898

(Clinical Cancer Center)

Nebraska

University of Nebraska Medical Center/

Eppley Cancer Center

600 South 42nd Street

Omaha, NE 68198-6805

Phone (402) 559-4238; fax (402) 559-4652

(Clinical Cancer Center)

New Hampshire

Norris Cotton Cancer Center

Dartmouth-Hitchcock Medical Center

One Medical Center Drive

Lebanon, NH 03756-0001

Phone (603) 653-9000; fax (603) 653-9003

(Comprehensive Cancer Center)

New Jersey

Cancer Institute of New Jersey

Robert Wood Johnson University Hospital

Robert Wood Johnson Medical School
195 Little Albany Street, Room 2002B
New Brunswick, NJ 08901
Phone (732) 235-8064; fax (732) 235-8094
(Comprehensive Cancer Center)

New York
Cancer Research Center
Albert Einstein College of Medicine
Chanin Building, Room 209
1300 Morris Park Avenue
Bronx, NY 10461
Phone (718) 430-2302; fax (718) 430-8550
(Clinical Cancer Center)

Roswell Park Cancer Institute
Elm and Carlton Streets
Buffalo, NY 14263-0001
Phone (716) 845-5772; fax (716) 845-8261
(Comprehensive Cancer Center)

Cold Spring Harbor Laboratory
PO Box 100
Cold Spring Harbor, NY 11724
Phone (516) 367-8383; fax (516) 367-8879
(Cancer Center)

NYU Cancer Institute
New York University Medical Center
550 First Avenue
New York, NY 10016
Phone (212) 263-8950; fax (212) 263-8210
(Clinical Cancer Center)

Memorial Sloan-Kettering Cancer Center
1275 York Avenue
New York, NY 10021
Phone (212) 639-2000, (800) 525-2225; fax (212) 717-3299
(Comprehensive Cancer Center)

Institute for Cancer Prevention
390 Fifth Avenue, 3rd Floor
New York, NY 10018
Phone (212) 551-2500; fax (212) 687-2339
(Cancer Center)

Herbert Irving Comprehensive Cancer Center
College of Physicians and Surgeons
Columbia University
161 Fort Washington Avenue
11th Floor, Room 1153
New York, NY 10032
Phone (212) 305-5201; fax (212) 305-6813
(Comprehensive Cancer Center)

North Carolina
UNC Lineberger Comprehensive Cancer Center
University of North Carolina, Chapel Hill
School of Medicine, CB-7295
102 West Drive
Chapel Hill, NC 27599-7295
Phone (919) 966-3036; fax (919) 966-3015
(Comprehensive Cancer Center)

Duke Comprehensive Cancer Center
Duke University Medical Center
Box 3843

Durham, NC 27710
Phone (919) 684-5613; fax (919) 684-5653
(Comprehensive Cancer Center)

Comprehensive Cancer Center
Wake Forest University
Medical Center Boulevard
Winston-Salem, NC 27157-1082
Phone (336) 716-7971; fax (336) 716-0293
(Comprehensive Cancer Center)

Ohio
Ireland Cancer Center
Case Western Reserve University and
University Hospitals of Cleveland
11100 Euclid Avenue, Wearn 151
Cleveland, OH 44106-5065
Phone (216) 844-8562; fax (216) 844-4975
(Comprehensive Cancer Center)

Comprehensive Cancer Center
Arthur G. James Cancer Hospital and
Richard J. Solove Research Institute
Ohio State University
A458 Staring Loving Hall
320 West 10th Avenue
Columbus, OH 43210
Phone (614) 293-7521; fax (614) 293-7522
(Comprehensive Cancer Center)

Oregon
OHSU Cancer Institute
Oregon Health and Science University

3181 SW Sam Jackson Park Road, CR145
Portland, OR 97201-3098
Phone (503) 494-1617; fax (503) 494-7086
(Clinical Cancer Center)

Pennsylvania
Abramson Cancer Center
University of Pennsylvania
16th Floor, Penn Tower
3400 Spruce Street
Philadelphia, PA 19104-4283
Phone (215) 662-6065; fax (215) 349-5325
(Comprehensive Cancer Center)

Wistar Institute
3601 Spruce Street
Philadelphia, PA 19104-4268
Phone (215) 898-3926; fax (215) 573-2097
(Cancer Center)

Fox Chase Cancer Center
7701 Burholme Avenue
Philadelphia, PA 19111
Phone (215) 728-2781; fax (215) 728-2571
(Comprehensive Cancer Center)

Kimmel Cancer Center
Thomas Jefferson University
233 South 10th Street
BLSB, Room 1050
Philadelphia, PA 19107-5799
Phone (215) 503-4645; fax (215) 923-3528
(Clinical Cancer Center)

University of Pittsburgh Cancer Institute
UPMC Cancer Pavilion
5150 Centre Avenue, Suite 500
Pittsburgh, PA 15232
Phone (412) 623-3205; fax (412) 623-3210
(Comprehensive Cancer Center)

Tennessee
St. Jude Children's Research Hospital
332 North Lauderdale
PO Box 318
Memphis, TN 38105-2794
Phone (901) 495-3301; fax (901) 525-2720
(Clinical Cancer Center)

Vanderbilt-Ingram Cancer Center
Vanderbilt University
691 Preston Research Building
Nashville, TN 37232-6838
Phone (615) 936-1782; fax (615) 936-1790
(Comprehensive Cancer Center)

Texas
M. D. Anderson Cancer Center
University of Texas
1515 Holcombe Boulevard, Box 91
Houston, TX 77030
Phone (713) 792-2121; fax (713) 799-2210
(Comprehensive Cancer Center)

San Antonio Cancer Institute
University of Texas Health Science Center
Department of Hematology

7703 Floyd Curl Drive
San Antonio, TX 78229-3900
Phone (210) 567-4848; fax (210) 567-1956
(Clinical Cancer Center)

Utah
Huntsman Cancer Institute
University of Utah
2000 Circle of Hope
Salt Lake City, UT 84112-5550
Phone (801) 585-3401; fax (801) 585-6345
(Clinical Cancer Center)

Vermont
Vermont Cancer Center
University of Vermont
149 Beaumont Avenue, HRSF326
Burlington, VT 05405
Phone (802) 656-4414; fax (802) 656-8788
(Comprehensive Cancer Center)

Virginia
Cancer Center
University of Virginia, Health Sciences Center
Jefferson Park Avenue, Room 617E
Charlottesville, VA 22908
Phone (434) 243-9926; fax (434) 982-0918
(Clinical Cancer Center)

Massey Cancer Center
Virginia Commonwealth University
PO Box 980037

Richmond, VA 23298-0037
Phone (804) 828-0450; fax (804) 828-8453
(Clinical Cancer Center)

Washington
Fred Hutchinson Cancer Research Center
PO Box 19024, D1-060
Seattle, WA 98109-1024
Phone (206) 667-4305; fax (206) 667-5268
(Comprehensive Cancer Center)

Wisconsin
Comprehensive Cancer Center
University of Wisconsin
600 Highland Avenue, Room K4/610
Madison, WI 53792-0001
Phone (608) 263-8610; fax (608) 263-8613
(Comprehensive Cancer Center)

Index

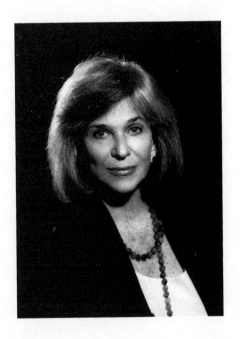

Ruth H. Grobstein, M.D., Ph.D.,
is founding director of the Ida M.
and Cecil H. Green Cancer Center
and founding head of radiation
oncology at the Scripps Clinic in
San Diego, where she also holds
the Rosenthal Chair in Cancer
Prevention and Screening.

Tear-Out Decision Trees

Decision Tree 1A How to Proceed If You Find a New Lump in Your Breast

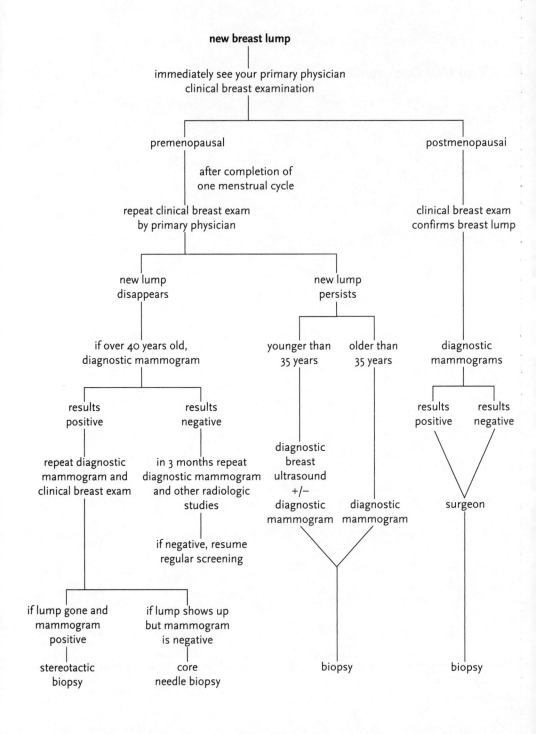

Decision Tree 1B How to Proceed If You Don't Find a New Breast Lump
(Regular Breast Screening)

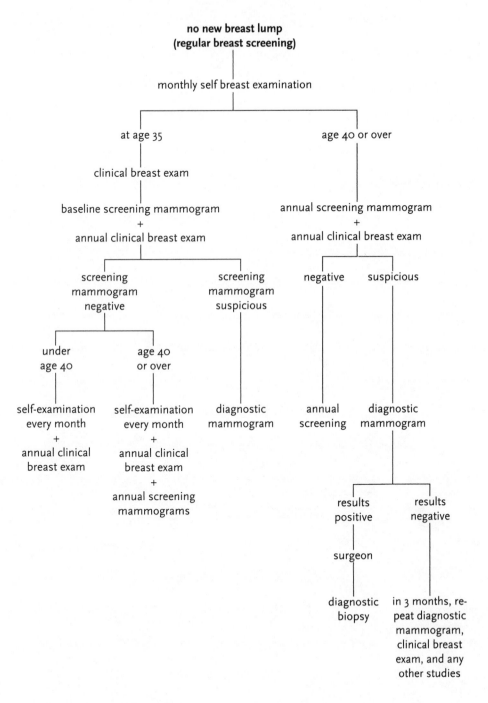

Decision Tree 2 When Your Screening Mammogram
Is Suspicious

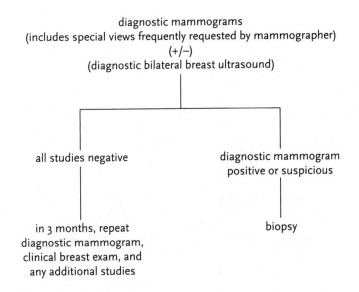

diagnostic mammograms
(includes special views frequently requested by mammographer)
(+/−)
(diagnostic bilateral breast ultrasound)

all studies negative

diagnostic mammogram
positive or suspicious

in 3 months, repeat
diagnostic mammogram,
clinical breast exam, and
any additional studies

biopsy

Decision Tree 3 Breast Biopsies

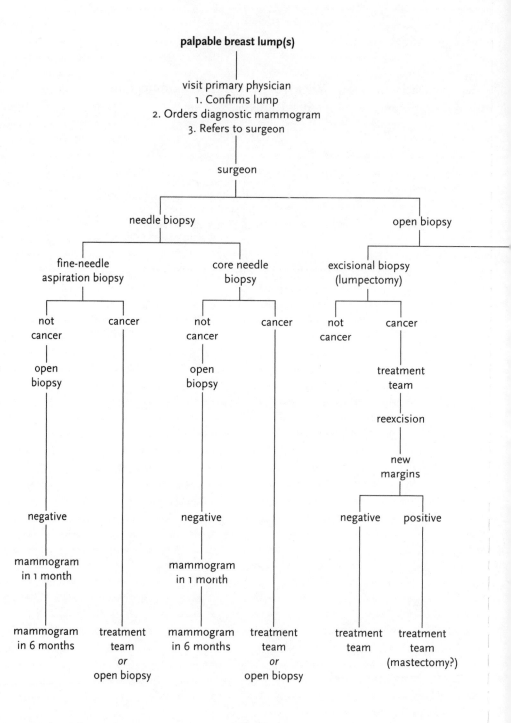

palpable breast lump(s)

visit primary physician
1. Confirms lump
2. Orders diagnostic mammogram
3. Refers to surgeon

surgeon

needle biopsy   open biopsy

fine-needle
aspiration biopsy   core needle
biopsy   excisional biopsy
(lumpectomy)

not
cancer   cancer   not
cancer   cancer   not
cancer   cancer

open
biopsy   open
biopsy   treatment
team

reexcision

new
margins

negative   negative   negative   positive

mammogram
in 1 month   mammogram
in 1 month

mammogram
in 6 months   treatment
team
or
open biopsy   mammogram
in 6 months   treatment
team
or
open biopsy   treatment
team   treatment
team
(mastectomy?)

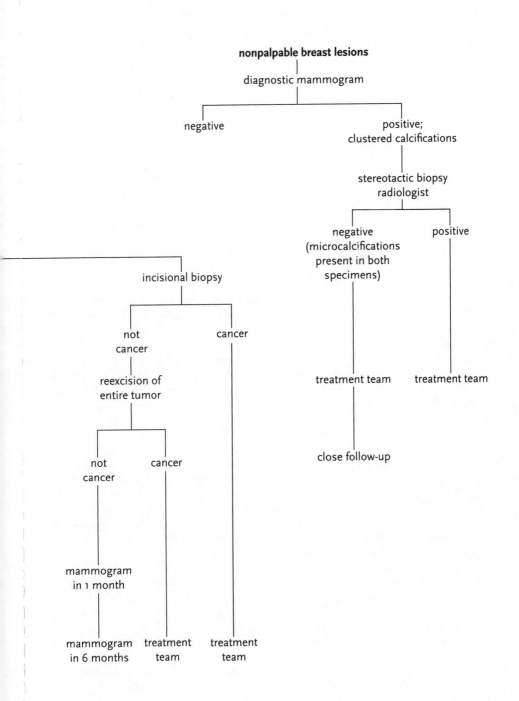

Decision Tree 4 The Treatment Team

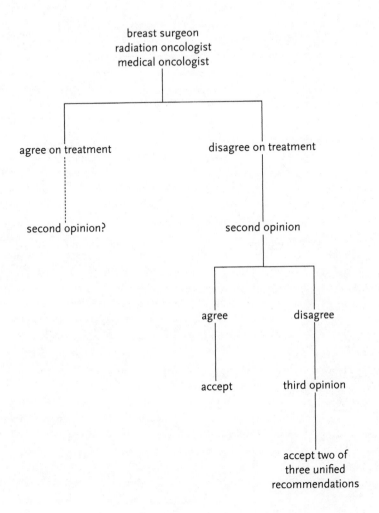

Decision Tree 5 Surgical Options

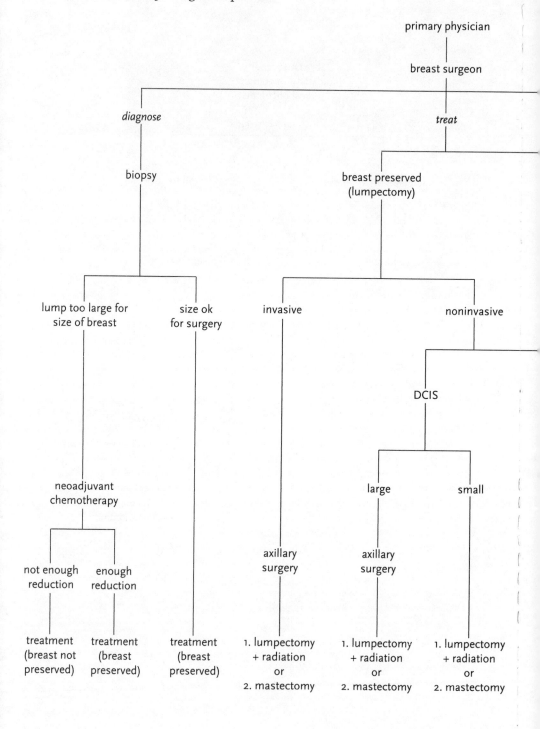

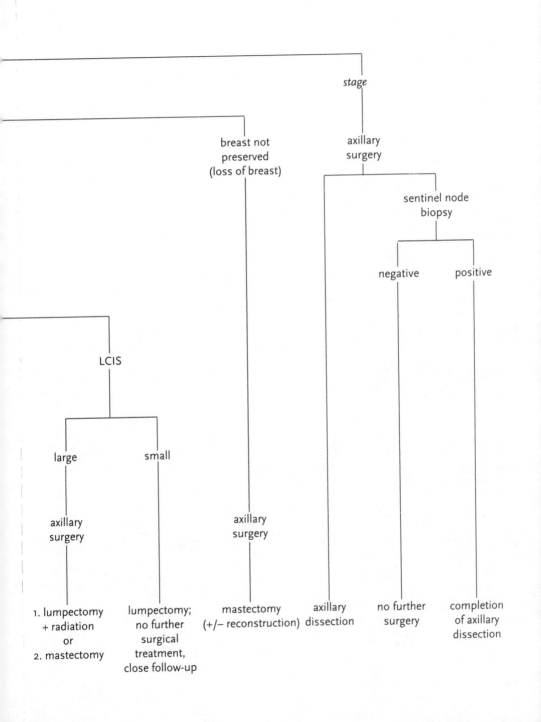

stage

breast not
preserved
(loss of breast)

axillary
surgery

sentinel node
biopsy

negative   positive

LCIS

large   small

axillary
surgery

axillary
surgery

1. lumpectomy   lumpectomy;   mastectomy   axillary   no further   completion
   + radiation   no further   (+/− reconstruction) dissection   surgery   of axillary
   or   surgical   dissection
2. mastectomy   treatment,
                  close follow-up

Decision Tree 6 Radiation

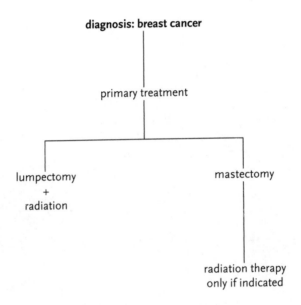

diagnosis: breast cancer

primary treatment

lumpectomy
+
radiation

mastectomy

radiation therapy
only if indicated

Decision Tree 7 Systemic Therapy

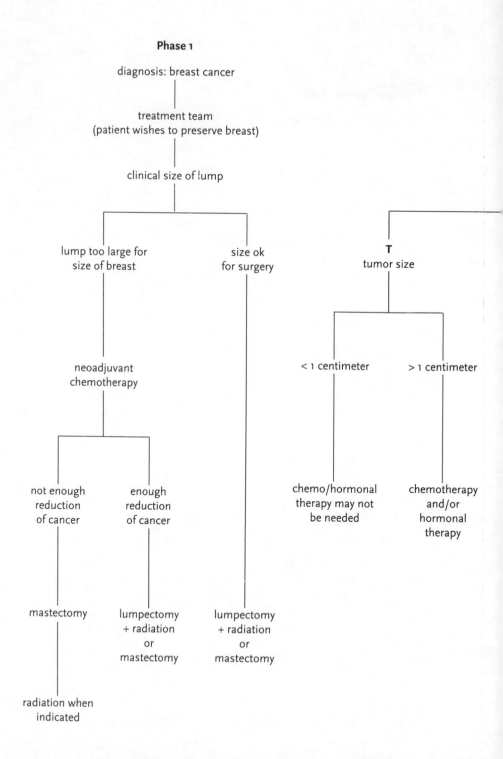

Phase 1

diagnosis: breast cancer

treatment team
(patient wishes to preserve breast)

clinical size of lump

lump too large for
size of breast

size ok
for surgery

T
tumor size

neoadjuvant
chemotherapy

< 1 centimeter

> 1 centimeter

not enough
reduction
of cancer

enough
reduction
of cancer

chemo/hormonal
therapy may not
be needed

chemotherapy
and/or
hormonal
therapy

mastectomy

lumpectomy
+ radiation
or
mastectomy

lumpectomy
+ radiation
or
mastectomy

radiation when
indicated

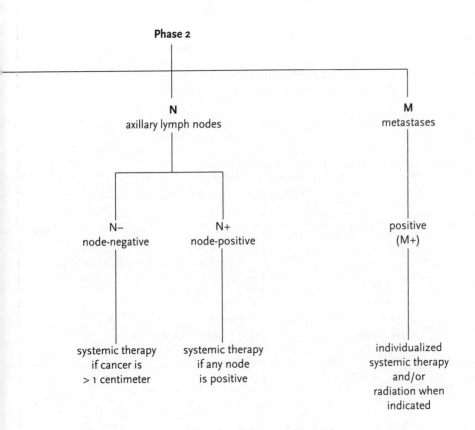

Phase 2

N
axillary lymph nodes

M
metastases

N–
node-negative

N+
node-positive

positive
(M+)

systemic therapy
if cancer is
> 1 centimeter

systemic therapy
if any node
is positive

individualized
systemic therapy
and/or
radiation when
indicated

Decision Tree 8 Return Visits after Treatment Is Finished

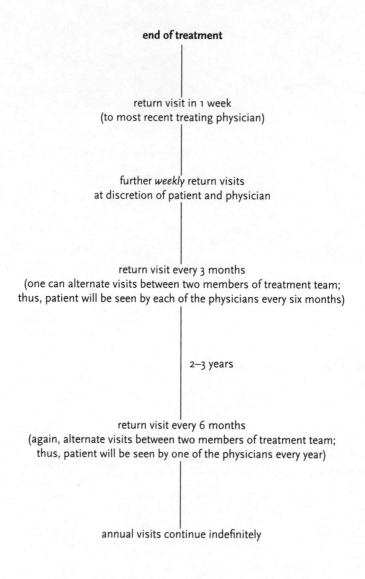

end of treatment

return visit in 1 week
(to most recent treating physician)

further *weekly* return visits
at discretion of patient and physician

return visit every 3 months
(one can alternate visits between two members of treatment team;
thus, patient will be seen by each of the physicians every six months)

2–3 years

return visit every 6 months
(again, alternate visits between two members of treatment team;
thus, patient will be seen by one of the physicians every year)

annual visits continue indefinitely